SPORTS SUPPLEMENT BUYER'S GUIDE

Complete Nutrition for Your Active Lifestyle

Stephen Adelé
& Rehan Jalali

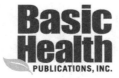

Basic Health
PUBLICATIONS, INC.

The information contained in this book is based upon the research and personal and professional experiences of the authors. It is not intended as a substitute for consulting with your physician or other healthcare provider. Any attempt to diagnose and treat an illness should be done under the direction of a healthcare professional.

The publisher does not advocate the use of any particular healthcare protocol but believes the information in this book should be available to the public. The publisher and authors are not responsible for any adverse effects or consequences resulting from the use of the suggestions, preparations, or procedures discussed in this book. Should the reader have any questions concerning the appropriateness of any procedures or preparation mentioned, the authors and the publisher strongly suggest consulting a professional healthcare advisor.

Stephen Adelé, the coauthor of this book, has a financial interest in iSatori products. This does not constitute an endorsement by Basic Health Publications, Inc.

Basic Health Publications, Inc.
28812 Top of the World Drive
Laguna Beach, CA 92651
949-715-7327 • www.basichealthpub.com

Library of Congress Cataloging-in-Publication Data

Adelé, Stephen.
   Sports supplement buyer's guide : complete nutrition for your active lifestyle / Stephen Adelé and Rehan Jalali.
      p. cm.
   Includes bibliographical references and index.
   ISBN 978-1-59120-166-3
   1. Dietary supplements. 2. Athletes—Nutrition. I. Jalali, Rehan. II. Title.

   RM258.5.A34   2007
   615'.1—dc22

                                                                    2007009683

Editor: John Anderson
Typesetting/Book design: Gary A. Rosenberg
Cover design: Mike Stromberg

Printed in the United States of America

10 9 8 7 6 5 4 3 2 1

Contents

Introduction

Whether you're a professional athlete, hardcore weight lifter, sports enthusiast, or just beginning to work out, you've probably thought about using supplements to enhance your training or recover from injuries. But one look at the supplement section at the local health food store or at your gym may have caused second thoughts. There are so many sports supplements available on the market today: tubs of protein powders, energy bars, amino acids for muscle building, fat-burner nutrients, and so on. You may have wondered, Do I really need to take supplements? Which ones should I take? And how do I know the good ones from the not-so-good ones?

First of all, if you're active in sports or exercise, you should probably consider taking dietary supplements. A dietary supplement provides nutrients (such as a vitamins or minerals) that are low or missing from a person's diet. Part of the name says it all—a "supplement" is something that is added to the diet or supplements a diet. In other words, a supplement doesn't replace the diet totally but has an additive or supraphysiological effect. Dietary supplements are not magic bullets or lightning in a bottle that will miraculously cure all your ailments and give you the body of your dreams. It takes a combination of good nutrition, hard training, and motivation, along with dietary supplements, to do that.

Official Definition of a Dietary Supplement

In the United States, a dietary supplement is defined under the Dietary Supplement Health and Education Act (DSHEA) of 1994 as a product that meets each of the following criteria:

1. It is intended to supplement the diet and bears or contains one or more of the following dietary ingredients:
   - Vitamin
   - Mineral
   - Herb or other botanical (excluding tobacco)
   - Amino acid
   - A dietary substance for use by man to supplement the diet by increasing the total daily intake (e.g., enzymes or tissues from organs or glands)
   - A concentrate, such as a meal replacement or energy bar
   - Metabolite, constituent, or extract

2. It is intended for ingestion in pill, capsule, tablet, or liquid form.

3. It is not represented for use as a conventional food or as the sole item of a meal or diet.

4. It is labeled as a "dietary supplement."

The U.S. Food and Drug Administration (FDA) does not regulate dietary supplements like it does drugs—there is no burden of pre-approval of dietary supplements for safety or efficacy as there is for drugs. But contrary to popular belief, the FDA has full authority to remove a product from the market if it deems it to be unsafe. This happened in the case of the herbal fat-burner *ephedra*. In many ways, the FDA looks at dietary supplements as foods.

Dietary Supplements vs. Drugs

What is the difference between drugs and dietary supplements? There are plenty. First of all, drugs are synthetic, chemically created molecules that have powerful effects in the body (not to mention side effects). Dietary supplements are more natural and may be found in the food supply. They can be safely used at certain doses to have solid physiological effects. Next, drugs take years to come out and are stringently regulated by the FDA, while dietary supplements can be launched rather quickly in comparison. Have you ever seen those drug commercials where the guy blurts out a bunch of side effects that have occurred with the drug at the end? Well, that is certainly an issue with prescription medicines due to their powerful nature. One obvious difference is that you need to go to a doctor to get a prescription drug—this can be expensive and time consuming. In contrast, you can get a dietary supplement at a health food or grocery store—they are convenient and cost effective.

Recently, due to the prohormone/prosteroid nutrients, the line between drug and dietary supplements has been blurred. In fact, some dietary supplement herbs are standardized for drug-like compounds. In other words, they may have the same physiological mechanism of action as a prescription medicine. For example, the herb *St. John's wort* has been tested for depression (some studies actually compared it to prescription drugs). The nutrient nexrutine can inhibit cyclooxygenase-2 (COX-2) enzymes, producing anti-inflammatory effects like some prescription drugs. But since it's part of the whole herb, it may be safer yet potent. It is important to look at the dosages and quality of manufacturing/manufacturers.

Safe, Research-Based, Effective, and Easy to Use

"Don't Believe the Hype" was a popular song by the rap group Public Enemy, but judging by the hype out there giving dietary supplements a bad name, a lot of marketing people didn't listen to it. These "snake oil" salesmen have created a lot of skeptics regarding dietary supplements. But the fact is that dietary supplements have volumes of research behind them. Do a search on Medline, a government database of published research studies available on the Internet (www.pubmed.com) for vitamin C or creatine and you will find hundreds of clinical studies verifying their effective use in humans.

Actually, reputable supplement companies also perform research studies on their specific products, and many of these studies are published in peer-reviewed scientific journals. Gone are the days of throwing some pills in a bottle and selling them out of the garage—nowadays, dietary supplements are more "drug-like" when it comes to research testing. Credible companies know the liabilities associated with low quality or untested products, so they take the time and spend the money to get clinical studies done. In fact, there are organizations that specialize in performing clinical testing on dietary supplements specifically. There are also self-imposed GMPs (good manufacturing practices) and certifications like cGMP (current good manufacturing practices) that demonstrate the level of quality for the manufacturing of a dietary supplement.

The bottom line is that there are many dietary supplements that are safe, research-based, effective, and easy to use. They can be an important part of staying fit and active, so that you can keep enjoying your favorite sport or activity indefinitely. We'll help you sort through the array of sports supplements available and help you come up with a supplement regime to fit your specific needs and goals.

Integrated Supplementation for Maximum Impact

There are many reasons to take dietary supplements. For the active person and sports enthusiast, it is vital to maintain good nutrient intake. Also, dietary supplements can help recovery from injuries, promote the health of specific body systems, and be used for training goals, such as building muscle mass or burning body fat.

Every strong structure has a solid foundation. Without a good base, most buildings would collapse. The same can be said for your body. If you provide it with the basics, then it can grow strong and lean. It is extremely important to consume the basic building blocks when it comes to supplements to truly have success in your training program or sport. The base of the supplement pyramid must be strong to build the rest of it.

Top athletes such as quarterback Brett Favre and former NBA star Michael Jordan started with fundamental skills and took them to a very high level. Without the base skills, they would not be successful. If you are training hard and eating smart, then taking certain supplements can help you get better results quicker. But you must start with the basics before you can reap all the benefits of the advanced supplements. Once the basics are in place, then you can start integrating essential and advanced supplements to take your results to the next level.

Foundation Supplements

One obvious reason to supplement is to prevent any nutritional deficiencies and "food type" supplements can help. No one can eat a perfect food diet day in and day out for years. Especially with our busy lives and eating on the go, and the degradation of our food supply (due to environmental pollutants, food manufacturing changes, and other factors), many of us will have basic nutritional deficiencies. This problem is compounded if we exercise consistently or are under stress.

Nutrients such as protein and carbohydrates fit into this category. Protein is the key building block of lean muscle. Since getting a good dose of protein daily from food in our hectic lives is nearly impossible, protein supplements can save the day. They come in various forms including pure protein powders, meal replacement powders (MRPs), crackers, chips, and ready-to-drink shakes. One of the keys to getting a great body and maintaining strength is eating small, frequent meals daily. But our often hectic lives make it nearly impossible to get all these meals. This is where MRPs and high-protein nutrition bars can really help. You must make sure you are consuming plenty of protein as a base before moving on to more advanced supplements.

Carbohydrates are important for supporting energy levels, sparing muscle protein, and enhancing muscle hydration. Low-carbohydrate diets have been popular, but for athletes it is absolutely necessary to get the appropriate amount and type of carbohydrates to maximize performance.

Essential Supplements

Essential supplements act as a nutrient safety net and lower the chances of specific nutrient deficiencies. Nutrients like vitamins and minerals fit into this category. Exercising individuals need higher levels of these basic nutrients and it is not feasible to get them all through food alone. I believe there should be a new standard for vitamins and minerals that takes into account the needs of hard-training athletes. The Recommended Dietary Intake for Athletes (RDIA) sets a higher standard that we feel will appropriately address the needs of athletes.

Another example is essential fatty acids (EFAs)—since your body cannot produce them endogenously, supplementation is a great way to take in these essential nutrients. Antioxidants, which are nutrients that help destroy free radicals (damaging compounds), also belong in this category, since they may be very beneficial to exercising individuals. Antioxidants, such as vitamins C and E, N-acetylcysteine, and zinc, can help delay muscle fatigue, help keep athletes from getting sick by boosting immune function (you can't train while you're sick!), and allow for better recovery from exercise.

Amino acids are the building blocks or components of proteins. An example is BCAAs (branched-chain amino acids). BCAAs can be found in foods, but supplementation is the only way to get research-proven amounts of these amino acids. Consuming higher amounts of BCAAs increases lean muscle mass and decreases muscle breakdown.

Performance Supplements

Performance supplements are highly advanced and specific supplements designed to maximize physical and mental performance. Some dietary supplements can be taken for specific, targeted effects. In other words, they address one desired area of improvement, including the following targeted effects:

- Fat loss

- Muscle building

- Increased energy and endurance

- Insulin management and controlling blood sugar

- Blocking the stress hormone cortisol

- Boosting the hormones testosterone and human growth hormone

- Joint health and repair

For example, there are specific nutrients that can help joint health (glucosamine), enhance brain function (the herb *Ginkgo biloba*), or even enhance sleep (melatonin). Other supplements like creatine or beta-alanine can directly improve exercise performance, strength, and lean muscle mass.

There are also conditionally specific dietary supplements. These are supplements taken during certain times only, not all the time. For example, many people take extra vitamin C or the herb *echinacea* when they get a cold or the flu. Other nutrients like *Rhodiola rosea* are good to take during times of intense stress. There are also some supplements that can be very beneficial during hardcore dieting and intense sports or fitness training (like phosphatidylserine).

Putting It All Together

This book presents a rational plan for putting together a supplementation plan for athletes integrating all of these levels. I truly believe it takes a combination of each of these levels of supplementation to achieve maximum results from a fitness program. These levels also help fitness enthusiasts at different points in their routines. For example, a beginner may only want to take foundation supplements to start, while someone more advanced may want to take supplements from all three levels.

Like anything else, you need to work your way up to each level. It also depends on the goal and individual situation of the athlete. An injured athlete who is recovering from injury may actually need a supplement from each category to heal faster, even though he may not be an advanced athlete. What you will find in this book is detailed information on supplements that fit into each of the three levels (foundation, essential, and performance). Armed with this powerful information, you can become a much more educated consumer and choose supplements to help you safely and effectively achieve your goals. Results is what it's all about!

LEVEL 1

Foundation

The Importance of Whole Foods

To build your best body ever, it takes a combination of proper nutrition, training, and supplementation, with nutrition being the most important of the three. Athletes need to make sure that healthy food is the base of their program. Remember, supplements are exactly what their name implies, a supplement to a good eating program. Healthy nutrition comes first, then you can incorporate sports supplements. Whole foods provide protein, carbohydrates (including sugar and fiber), and fat (including saturated, unsaturated, and essential fatty acids).

Protein

Protein is one of the key macronutrients, along with carbohydrates and fats. It is the building block of muscle and amino acids are the building blocks of protein. Protein provides 4 calories per gram. There are essential amino acids, ones you must get from the diet because your body cannot produce them (tryptophan, lysine, methionine, phenylalanine, threonine, valine, leucine, and isoleucine), and non-essential amino acids (such as tyrosine, glycine, cysteine, proline, serine, and aspartic acid).

Branched-chain amino acids (BCAAs), which include L-leucine, L-isoleucince, and L-valine, are special amino acids that are very important for athletes because they may enhance athletic performance, increase lean body mass, and support the recovery process.

Protein has many benefits to someone who is exercising and even to sedentary individuals. It has been shown to increase lean body mass, enhance immune function, lower muscle breakdown secondary to weight training, and even increase strength. One of the primary uses of protein in the body is to synthesize structural proteins such as muscle, skin, and hair. Protein is also used to synthesize peptide hormones such as growth hormone (GH), insulin-like growth factor 1 (IGF-1), and insulin. Additionally, protein is used to synthesize key enzymes and other transport proteins essential to normal bodily function.

Most people cannot consume the amount of protein from whole foods that is necessary for optimal body function when involved in weight training or an exercise regimen—but they should at least try. Studies have shown that individuals who exercise have a much greater protein requirement than sedentary individuals. I would recommend that hard-training athletes and fitness enthusiasts consume at least 1 gram of protein per pound of bodyweight. So if you weigh 150 pounds, you would consume 150 grams of protein per day (preferably divided into 5–6 small meals).

Vegetarians can get protein from soy protein isolate or egg albumin (egg whites), or dairy if they are lacto ovo vegetarians and not vegans.

Top Food Protein Choices

Egg Whites. This protein is the "regular old Joe" protein and boasts a great amino acid profile.

Chicken Breast. Chicken is a relatively low-fat, high-quality protein source. It contains fairly high doses of BCAAs and has a good potassium to sodium ratio (which can positively influence water balance). For those who just can't eat chicken, turkey breast is a reasonable alternative.

Top Sirloin Steak. Sirloin is a lean protein source with an excellent potassium to sodium ratio. It provides iron and good amounts of the amino acids alanine and lysine. Make sure to ask the butcher to trim away all the visible fat. Other lean cuts of beef include top round steak and eye of round.

Tuna. Tuna is another lean protein source that provides an excellent amount of BCAAs. Canned versions make it easy to use and help with portion control.

Orange Roughy Fish. Orange roughy is a very lean protein source with an outstanding potassium to sodium ratio. It is a good source of the amino acids leucine and lysine. Other good fish include halibut, sea bass, mahi mahi, tilapia, cold-water salmon (not farmed, but wild), and ahi tuna.

Skim Milk. Skim milk is a solid protein source providing milk protein, which contains casein, a slow-release protein. It has a good amount of the amino acid L-leucine and also a decent amount of potassium. Since it contains calcium, it may also support healthy bones. Choose skim milk to skip out on the excess fat of regular or low-fat milk. Soy milk can be a good alternative for women, but for men it may be too estrogenic.

Carbohydrates

Carbohydrates are the major source of energy for most humans, providing 4 calories per gram. There are various types of carbohydrates, such as simple sugars, complex carbohydrates, and dietary fiber. Simple sugars are rapidly broken down and absorbed by the body, while complex carbs are more slowly digested and absorbed. Carbohydrates to avoid include sucrose, high-fructose corn syrup, and processed carbs like instant white rice and white bread.

The glycemic index is a rating of carbohydrates and their effect on blood sugar levels. The higher the glycemic index of a certain carbohydrate, the greater the blood sugar response after eating it. High blood sugar responses to foods can cause fat storage to occur and cause "yo-yo" energy levels. Consuming dietary fiber can lower the glycemic effect of carbohydrates. Carbohydrates are stored in the body as glycogen in the liver and in muscle tissue. Eating lower glycemic index carbohydrates can allow for a steady release of energy and help keep blood sugar levels stable.

Fruit is very interesting in that it provides a form of carbohydrate called fructose. This is a low-glycemic carbohydrate, but since it is metabolized primarily in the liver, it can slow down metabolism and may cause fat storage to occur if eaten in excess. So, fruit is fine for hard-training athletes but if you're trying to get really lean, you may want to limit it's consumption.

Lower-glycemic carbohydrates like sweet potatoes and multi-grain oatmeal are good carbs. The more processed and instantized a food is (thereby increasing its entrance into the bloodstream), the higher its glycemic index. For example, slow-cooked rice has a lower glycemic rating than instant rice. But as good as the glycemic index is for rating the effects of carbohydrates on blood sugar levels, it is deficient in that it doesn't address the issue of mixed meals. In other words, when someone eats a mixed meal containing protein along with carbohydrates (such as a tuna sandwich), the glycemic (and hence blood sugar) response will be much lower. The same is true for mixing carbohydrates with fat or dietary fiber. A more comprehensive scale would be a mixed meals glycemic scale.

The bottom line is that athletes need to consume plenty of good carbs to avoid "bonking." In the list of good carbohydrates, recommended carbs can be chosen from the first two columns, "complex" and "fibrous." Simple carbs (the third column) should only be eaen immediately following exercise, when the body can handle them.

Good Carbohydrates

Complex	Fibrous	Simple*
Oatmeal	Asparagus	Dates
Multi-grain oatmeal	Broccoli	Raisins
Yam	Cabbage	Grapefruit
Sweet potato	Cauliflower	Banana
White rice	Corn	Apple juice
Brown rice	Green Beans	Blueberries
Black beans	Tomato	Honey (unfiltered)
White potato	Lettuce	Apples
Whole-wheat pasta		

* Simple carbohydrates should only be eaten immediately post exercise.

Fiber

During the last twenty-five years, research has implicated dietary fiber as important in various aspects of gastrointestinal function and in supporting optimal health and weight reduction. Effects of fiber include increased fecal bulk, decreased luminal pressure, feeling full longer to control appetite, lowering the risk for colon cancer, delayed gastric emptying, lowering cholesterol, reduced glucose absorption (lowers glycemic index of foods), fat loss, and anti-toxic effects. Both soluble and insoluble fibers as well as "friendly" intestinal bacteria (probiotics) help support proper digestion and absorption of foods. The National Cancer Institute recommends 20–30 grams of fiber per day. FiberTeq from VPX Sports is a great fiber supplement.

Fats

I know it sounds strange, but there are actually many benefits to consuming fats for exercising individuals and athletes. Fat provides 9 calories per gram. Fats provide energy to the body and essential fats can help support hormone levels, neurological function, and cell membrane stability.

There are saturated and unsaturated fats. Saturated fats are the ones you generally want to avoid because of their detrimental effects in the body, such as cardiovascular problems (heart disease and increased cholesterol). These include trans-fats (partially hydrogenated and hydrogenated oils), animal fats, palm oil, and coconut oil. Unsaturated fats include the essential fatty acids (EFAs)—omega-3s (alpha-linolenic) and omega-6s (linoleic). These EFAs cannot be made by the body and must be taken in through foods or supplementation.

Some of the positive benefits of EFAs include: decreased catabolism and increased growth hormone secretion, improving the action of insulin, enhancing oxygen utilization and energy transformation required for optimal performance, decreasing total serum cholesterol and increasing HDL, improving testosterone production, supporting liver function and enhanced immune function, and improving the condition of hair and nails as well as increased nitrogen retention. These are all great effects for athletes or training individuals because these things may increase strength, support lean body mass, reduce body fat, and allow athletes to train harder and recover better from their workouts. A good product is Flax/Fish combination oil from Twinlab.

Quality Sources of Fats

- Fish oils (EPA and DHA)
- Flaxseed oil
- Olive or sunflower oils
- Peanut butter (all natural)
- Sunflower seeds (unsalted)
- Walnuts, almonds, or peanuts (unsalted)

SOME GENERAL RECOMMENDATIONS FOR SPECIFIC GOALS

Gaining Weight and Strength

To achieve this goal, it is important to eat more calories than you are expending. Limiting cardiovascular activity and performing mainly weight training is also helpful. Consume 16 calories per pound of body weight. For example, if you weigh 150 pounds, you will need to consume at least 2,400 calories daily, divided into 5–6 small meals throughout the day. You will need to eat a diet with a ratio of 50 percent carbohydrates, 25 percent protein, and 25 percent fat.

So, here's how it breaks down for a 150-pound person who requires 2,400 calories daily to gain weight:

- 50 percent carbohydrates = 2,400 ÷ 0.50 = 1,200 total calories from carbohydrates

  1,200 calories of carbs ÷ 4 calories per gram of carbs = 300 g of carbs daily

- 25 percent protein = 2,400 ÷ 0.25 = 600 total calories from protein daily

  600 calories of protein ÷ 4 calories per gram of protein = 150 g of protein daily

- 25 percent fat = 2,400 ÷ 0.25 = 600 total calories from fat daily

  600 calories of fat ÷ 9 calories per gram of fat = about 67 g of fat daily

Losing Weight and Toning

To lose body fat, it is important to consume less calories than you are expending daily. Avoiding simple sugars is beneficial. Try to eat smaller meals in the evening consisting of quality protein and fibrous carbohydrates (for example, a chicken breast and garden salad with non-fat dressing). Performing cardiovascular work (such as a brisk walk or bike ride) 3–4 times a week, preferably first thing in the morning, can be very helpful. Consume 10 calories per pound of body weight daily, with a daily food ratio of 45 percent protein, 40 percent carbohydrates, and 15 percent essential fats.

So, using the same calculations above, this equates to the following for a 150-pound person looking to lose weight:

- 1,500 daily calories

- 168 grams of protein

- 150 grams of carbohydrates

- 25 grams of essential fats

Building Muscle and Losing Fat

To gain muscle and lose fat, it is important to consume around 12 calories per pound of body weight daily. A good macronutrient ratio to follow is 40 percent protein, 40 percent carbohydrates, and 20 percent essential fat. This equates to the following for a 150-pound person:

- 1,800 daily calories

- 180 grams of protein

- 180 grams of carbohydrates

- 40 grams of essential fats

So, the moral of the story is to get your food intake in order first, then you can add in supplements to get better results!

Meal Replacement Powders and Shakes

Most of us know that quality nutrition and supplementation is the key to achieving athletic and physique success. It is important to eat 5–7 small meals daily to increase nutrient absorption, enhance metabolic rate, and help stabilize blood sugar (and insulin) levels. Eating small meals throughout the day makes logical sense, but it has also been shown to be beneficial according to clinical research. For example, a study published in the *Canadian Journal of Physiology and Pharmacology* showed that increased frequency of feeding helped stabilize insulin secretion. The researchers of this study went on to say that "increasing the number of meals increased thermogenesis and fat utilization." That sounds good to anyone looking to lose body fat! Yet another study states that increasing meal frequency can actually help lower LDL ("bad") cholesterol levels in normal people.

Convenience is always an issue in our busy lives. Meal replacement powders (MRPs) and the even more convenient ready-to-drink shakes allow you to get some of your meals in a convenient and generally tasty manner. (Who has the time to cook six meals daily?) They help improve overall nutrition and give you key nutrients your body needs to improve health and physical performance. Another great benefit to these products is they allow you to quantify exactly what you are consuming for that meal in terms or calories, protein, carbohydrates, and fat. This is important because daily caloric intake and the types of macronutrients consumed can go a long way in determining whether fat loss and/or lean muscle gain will be achieved. Unless you have a food scale and calorie count book with you wherever you go, it is hard to measure this with whole foods.

Most MRPs can be considered a complete meal as they usually contain protein, carbohydrates, fat, and vitamins and minerals. So-called low-carbohydrate MRPs are showing up on the market, but in many cases these are just protein powders in packets. There are also "light" versions of some MRPs mainly for women.

Proteins

MRPs usually start out with a "proprietary protein blend" with some cool and marketable name such as metamyobiocellaten. Protein is the building block of muscle and numerous studies show that athletes and exercising individuals require more protein than sedentary individuals. Some MRPs may have only one protein source such as whey protein isolate, but it is preferred to get a protein blend to utilize all the functional benefits of different proteins. Most MRPs or at least the proteins in them are "agglomerated" or instantized, which means they go through a process that makes them easier to mix in liquid (i.e., no blender necessary).

Whey. Quality whey protein (especially whey protein isolate) has benefits including providing intact immunoglobulins to support immune function, providing the highest concentration of BCAAs (branched-chain amino acids leucine, isoleucine, and valine, which play a key role in the muscle-building process), it has a high BV (biological value), which means it is readily absorbed and utilized by human muscle tissue, and it may even support IGF-1 levels. Whey also contains about 50 percent essential amino acids. Some research suggests that whey protein can stimulate the appetite control hormone CCK (cholecystokinin), thereby helping to suppress appetite. New research is showing us that whey protein can preserve lean muscle mass and bone health while dieting and may even stimulate abdominal fat loss directly. The minor downsides to whey are that it is lower in natural glutamine and arginine content, is less filling than other slower-absorbed proteins, and quality whey protein isolate with preserved microfractions is a bit pricier than other proteins. Nonetheless, the benefits of quality whey protein have been clinically proven to be outstanding. Designer Whey from Next Nutrition is a quality product.

Casein. Casein is another milk protein that seems to have a timed-release effect, as it forms a gel in the gut to slow the transit time of amino acids, which may enhance absorption. It has a very high natural glutamine content, most in the peptide form for better absorption (due to peptide transport systems in the digestive tract). Casein also has a high ratio of tyrosine to tryptophan, so it could be considered a stimulating protein as well. Milk protein isolate contains both whey and casein and it is a good source for these two proteins.

Soy. Soy protein isolate has been shown to enhance thyroid hormone output, which can increase metabolic rate to support fat loss. The isoflavones in soy have numerous health benefits including cholesterol-lowering and triglyceride-lowering effects. It contains an excellent ratio of glutamine, arginine, and the BCAAs. It is a fairly low-priced protein source but can have positive benefits for women mainly, but men as well.

Egg albumin. Egg albumin protein boasts a great amino acid profile but does not offer very many functional benefits. It is a little harder to mix in liquid.

   Bottom Line: Look for an MRP that has 30–50 grams of protein per serving from a blend of proteins, not just a single source. Look for the protein blend to list whey protein isolate as the first or second ingredient.

Carbohydrates

MRPs contain carbohydrates as well.

Maltodextrin. Typically, the main source used to be maltodextrin, which is a very low cost ingredient derived from corn. Although it is considered a complex carbohydrate and a glucose polymer, it has a very high glycemic index rating (a rating that determines how your blood sugar and hence insulin responds after ingesting carbohydrates). In fact, maltodextrin's rating on the glycemic scale is right up there with maltose, which is glucose plus glucose. That means it can cause a large insulin response, which would be beneficial after a weight-training workout but not beneficial at other times of the day (although the protein in MRPs helps balance this out in terms of blood sugar response).

Corn syrup solids. Corn syrup solids is another ingredient you'll see on MRP labels; it is derived from the enzyme hydrolysis of corn.

Fructose. Fructose is fruit sugar and is added to MRPs not only to provide a source of carbohydrates but also to sweeten the product, as it has a very sweet taste. It is mainly metabolized in the liver and may lead to fat storage. Watch out for high-fructose corn syrup.

Brown rice. Brown rice syrup and brown rice complex also are sometimes added to provide complex carbohydrates.

Other sources. Other carbohydrate sources to look for on MRP labels include oat bran fiber, whole grain brown rice, and inulin.

Some MRPs are also fortified with dietary fiber (one problem with many MRPs is they do not have a lot of fiber in them). During the last twenty years, research has implicated dietary fiber as important for gastrointestinal function and in the prevention of disease. Insoluble fibers include lignin, cellulose, and some hemicellulose. Soluble fibers include pectin, gum, mucilages, and some hemicellulose. Fiber increases fecal bulk, decreases luminal pressure, delays gastric emptying, reduces glucose absorption (lowers glycemic index of foods), prevents colon cancer, and eliminates toxins. Fiber makes an MRP thicker when mixed in solution.

Bottom Line: Look for an MRP that contains 15–35 grams of quality carbohydrates with at least 5 grams of fiber and less than 5 grams of sugar per serving.

Essential Fatty Acids

Essential fatty acids (EFAs) are also added to MRPs, including borage oil, sunflower oil, flaxseeds and flaxseed oil, MCTs (medium-chain triglycerides, which are listed as saturated fats on the label but act differently in the body), and primrose oil. EFAs have many benefits including improved metabolism, improved insulin action, increased growth hormone secretion, improved testosterone production, improved blood pressure, liver support and protection (especially with borage oil and evening primrose oil), improved condition of hair and nails, improved cholesterol profile, decreased inflammation response, improved nerve function, enhanced immune function, improved energy production of cells, and increased nitrogen retention.

Some "special fats" like CLA and SesaLean™ are also showing up in some MRPs. CLA is a "special fat" that has been shown to help with fat reduction and lean muscle mass gain (it can also help boost immune function). SesaLean™ is a special sesame oil extract that may support the fat-loss process.

Bottom Line: Look for an MRP to contain at least 4 grams of EFAs per serving and less than 2 grams of saturated fat. Look for special fats like CLA and sesame oil extract. Fat-free or low-fat MRPs are missing out on the benefits of EFAs.

Vitamins and Minerals

MRPs contain a blend of vitamins and minerals to support overall health and many chemical processes in the body. Vitamins and minerals are usually ancillary items to MRPs and many minerals in the formulas actually compete for absorption, like calcium and magnesium, plus they are usually not found in the higher absorbable chelated forms. Chromium is added to MRPs (usually in the better polynicotinate form) to support optimal blood sugar levels and help aid in fat loss. Also, many MRPs are higher in sodium, which may cause water retention to occur.

Bottom Line: It is good to look for an MRP that has at least a 2:1 (or better yet 3:1) ratio of potassium to sodium to optimize water balance. Don't worry too much about the vitamins and minerals in an MRP formula as they won't be enough to impact your program.

Other Ingredients

MRPs contain a lot unnecessary ingredients, including artificial colors (to make the product look palatable), hydrogenated oils (for "mouth feel"), and corn syrup solids and salt (for taste). MRPs are also sweetened with many different natural and artificial sweeteners, including sucralose (Splenda), acesulfame K, aspartame, stevia, and kiwi extract. Most of these sweeteners are calorie free or such a small amount is used that the calories are insufficient. Sucralose is 600 times sweeter than sugar and has been tested in over 100 studies showing safety and efficacy.

Aspartame seems to stir controversy as over 50 percent of the complaints the U.S. Food and Drug Administration (FDA) receives about food ingredients are related to aspartame. It is made up of the amino acids phenylalanine and aspartic acid along with methanol (wood alcohol). There is plenty of safety data behind it, but many individuals still seem to be sensitive to this sweetener. Individuals with PKU (a disorder in which the individual cannot metabolize phenylalanine), pregnant women, and nursing women should avoid aspartame.

Newer Formulas

Muscle Milk is a hugely popular product from CytoSport designed to deliver "metabolically favorable ingredients to stimulate growth and recovery in a similar manner to mother's milk" or so says their website. If you read the ingredient label, you'll be overwhelmed by the degree of "proprietary" ingredients and scientific jargon. This can be a convenient smokescreen when a company doesn't want you to know the ingredients in their products by common names, but sometimes it's also a sign of highly proprietary research and product development. Things like EvoPro, LEANLIPIDES, and Betapol are all trademarks for a host of nutrients including proteins and fats.

Another popular meal replacement protein shake is Eat-Smart® from iSatori Technologies. Eat-Smart is quite unique, because not only does it contain a good source of quality protein from whey isolate, but it's fortified with good carbs from oats, good fats from flaxseed, and added fiber, probiotics and enzymes to make it friendly on the stomach. What's really great about this product is that you can choose from an assortment of six great-tasting, dessert-like flavor enhancers to flavor it any way you want. You can find out more about it at www.eat-smartmrp.com.

Other quality MRPs include ZI Diet MRP from VPX Sports, Lean Body by Labrada, Myoplex Deluxe from EAS, and Eat-Smart from iSatori. So, check your nutrition plan, and make sure ready-to-drink products like these will fit into your caloric requirements.

Shakes

Although ready-to-drink (RTD) shakes are very convenient, the nutritional value is not as good as powders due to the process it takes to make them stable in liquid over time. Ready-to-drink shakes do not require the mixing that MRPs entail.

Bottom Line: RTD shakes can also be used as meal replacements, but their nutritional value will not be as good as MRP powders. Some good ones are Myoplex (which has various formulations, such as Lite and Carb Control™) by EAS, Lean Body by Labrada, and Nitro-Tech RTD by Muscle-Tech.

Dosage

Taking 1–3 MRP packets or RTD shakes daily to effectively replace meals can be beneficial as part of a complete nutrition and fitness program. Some of the best times to take these products are after a workout or first thing in the morning as a breakfast replacement (some companies like Labrada actual-ly have a specific breakfast MRP shake). Fresh (or frozen) fruit can be added, but keep in mind the extra calories. If you are looking to gain weight, then mixing them with skim milk may be beneficial. If you are looking to lose fat, then mix them with water (cold water works best to make them taste bet-ter, and adding ice can help).

Protein Powders and Nutrition Bars

Protein for an athlete or fitness enthusiast is absolutely vital. It is the base nutrient for building lean muscle as well as a host of other positive functions. Looking around at all the information (or misinformation) on protein, it's hard to decipher how to use protein to maximize all its benefits. The fact is that you must get adequate protein intake, otherwise you may be compromising your results.

Protein has many benefits to someone who is exercising and even to sedentary individuals. It has been shown to increase lean body mass, enhance immune function, lower muscle breakdown secondary to weight training, and it may even increase strength. One of the primary uses of protein in the body is to synthesize structural proteins such as muscle, skin, and hair. Protein is also used to synthesize peptide hormones such as growth hormone (GH), insulin-like growth factor 1 (IGF-1), and insulin. Proteins are made up of sub-units called amino acids. There are essential (your body cannot make these) and non-essential (your body can make these endogenously) amino acids.

Protein is a fundamental nutrient and therefore is vitally important for everyone to consume, which helps explain the popularity of protein powders and high-protein diets. Most people cannot consume the amount of protein from whole foods that is necessary for optimal body function when they are involved in weight training or an exercise regimen. Because individuals who exercise have a much greater protein requirement than sedentary individuals, protein powders can save the day. They are convenient, provide a good source of protein, may help suppress appetite, and they actually taste good, thanks to advanced flavor technologies.

The Top Protein Contenders
Whey Protein

Whey protein, a milk derivative, is by far the most popular protein on the market. Whey protein comes in various forms, such as concentrate and the better isolate form. The concentrate is a lower grade whey protein that does not provide the benefits of microfractions (active ingredients) and is usually higher in fat and lactose. Whey protein has a very high "biological value," which means it is readily utilized by human muscle tissue, thus making it a quickly absorbed protein (anabolic).

Advanced manufacturing procedures like cross-flow microfiltration lead to a higher quality whey with added benefits over ion-exchange whey isolate, preserving key microfractions that are essential to it's benefits. Whey protein isolate that is not heat-treated contains key microfractions such as alpha-lactalbumin and glycomacropeptides, which can both positively support immune function. Some growth factors found in whey protein can enhance IGF-1 levels, which can increase lean muscle mass—good news for training athletes! Most of the whey protein on the market is usually found as the ion-exchange (a process where electrical charges are used to extract the protein) form, and some users of whey protein concentrate may experience bloating or gas due to its lower quality.

Benefits: Quality whey protein isolate provides key microfractions, enhances glutathione levels in the body (glutathione is the body's most powerful natural antioxidant and is a key part of the immune system), features high digestibility and absorption rate, and contains virtually no lactose and very low fat. It also has a very high concentration of BCAAs (branched-chain amino acids), which can positively affect lean muscle mass and lower muscle breakdown (whey protein contains about 25 percent BCAAs—the highest of any protein source). Whey contains about 50 percent essential amino acids, which recent research has shown are vital for optimal muscle recovery and for supporting lean muscle mass. In fact, researchers report that pure whey protein may be more effective in increasing muscle mass and strength, while decreasing fat, compared to casein protein. New research shows that whey can help with fat loss (especially belly fat), preserve muscle while dieting, boost exercise performance, and even suppress appetite due to it's modification of CCK (cholecystokinin). CCK is a hormone that sends a signal to the brain to stop eating—it's known as a satiety hormone.

Downside: Whey protein is lower in natural glutamine and arginine content, is less filling than other more slowly absorbed proteins, and quality whey protein isolate with preserved microfractions is a bit pricier than other proteins.

Best Uses: Due to its quick absorption, whey protein is excellent to take before or even right after a hard workout. It also works as a between-meal snack for a protein boost in the middle of the day.

Casein

Casein is also a milk-derived protein and comes in various forms, including calcium caseinate, sodium caseinate, and micellar casein. Casein has a reputation for being the "anti-catabolic" (lowering muscle breakdown) protein and has some advantages over whey. First, casein is absorbed more slowly and can provide a sustained release of amino acids into the bloodstream over a longer period of time. It forms a gel in the stomach and the amino acids are extracted more slowly and may be better absorbed over the long run.

Studies confirm the benefits of casein over whey, showing casein's powerful ability to reduce muscle breakdown and increase protein synthesis. A recent study in police officers showed that the casein group lost more body fat, gained more lean muscle mass, and had greater strength increases than the whey protein group. The authors of the study attributed it to the anti-catabolic effects of the peptides (chains of amino acids) found naturally in casein. Peptides are absorbed better than amino acids due to peptide transport systems in the gut.

Benefits: Casein is more slowly absorbed, so there is a longer release of amino acids into the bloodstream and it has a very high glutamine content (especially in the better absorbed peptide form). Micellar casein (a higher quality form), which is undenatured (not heat-treated), contains some milk fractions that can boost immune function and increase growth factors in the body.

Downside: Casein has a higher lactose and sodium content, so water retention and some stomach discomfort could result.

Best Uses: As a pre-bedtime drink to lower muscle breakdown during sleep or for breakfast to provide a steady stream of amino acids in the morning.

Milk Protein Isolate

Milk protein isolate contains both whey and casein. This is a solid protein that gives you many of the benefits of both whey and casein.

Soy Protein Isolate (SPI)

Isolated soy protein has been the subject of many research studies and seems to be in the news a lot. It is a good protein source that has many positive health effects along with benefits to athletes. The Solae Company has a high-quality brand of isolated soy which is called Supro®, which you can find in many soy products on the market today. Even though many women use SPI, some newer studies support the use of SPI in training males.

One study in the *Journal of Nutrition* showed that soy protein increased IGF-1 (insulin-like growth factor-1) in young and old men. IGF-1 is a powerful muscle-building hormone that is responsible for many of the positive effects of growth hormone (GH), since GH converts to IGF-1 in the liver. Another study in the *European Journal of Clinical Nutrition* in 2003, and conducted at the University of Alabama at Birmingham, showed that a soy-based formula was effective in lowering body weight, body fat, and reduced low-density lipoprotein (LDL or "bad") cholesterol. A 2004 study conducted at the University of California—Los Angeles showed that a soy-based meal replacement enhanced weight loss and lowered C-reactive protein levels in type II diabetics (a measure of inflammation in the body and a risk factor for cardiovascular disease). Plus, it allowed the subjects to reduce their medications and helped with blood sugar control.

Some people have devalued the benefits of SPI as compared to whey protein, but researchers at Ohio State University published a study in the *Nutrition Journal* in 2004 and set the record straight. They compared the effects of whey and soy on lean muscle mass gain in weight-training males. The results showed that both the soy and whey protein had similar effects in promoting lean body mass. What's even more interesting is that only the soy protein group preserved two key aspects of antioxidant function, while the whey group showed a decrease in these factors post-training.

There has been a concern among males specifically that SPI may be estrogenic. However, recent research from Miami Research Associates presented at the 2005 FASEB conference in San Diego, California, debunks this theory. The researchers concluded that "daily supplementation of soy,

Protein Myths Exposed

Myth: Taking too much protein daily in healthy people can be damaging to the kidneys.

Fact: There are no research studies that show any adverse effect to the kidneys of healthy people when consuming higher levels of protein daily, even in excessive amounts. Excess protein that the body cannot use is broken down and eliminated or, in rare cases, is converted to fat. The only studies that show adverse effects to the kidneys with large intakes of protein daily are in people who have only one kidney. Again, exercising individuals need more protein. Note: For exercising individuals, it is important to drink plenty of water daily.

Myth: You can only absorb 30 grams of protein in one sitting.

Fact: The body has the ability to absorb and utilize more than 30 grams of protein per sitting. This varies from person to person, but research studies have used upwards of 40 grams of protein per sitting to stimulate muscle growth. Again, training athletes need plenty of protein to stimulate lean muscle mass and lower muscle breakdown. This requires that they consume more than 30 grams of protein in one sitting in many cases. By the way, most meal replacement powders on the market like Met-Rx and Myoplex have over 30 grams of protein per packet, yet many people use them effectively to gain muscle mass and lose body fat.

Myth: You should only take protein by itself and never take it with carbohydrates.

Fact: This couldn't be further from the truth. Combining protein with carbohydrates has several benefits. One is that the protein actually lowers the glycemic index, the rate at which the carbohydrate is absorbed, and thereby can reduce fat storage that may occur if the carbohydrate was consumed by itself (due to insulin release). Also, since carbohydrate intake stimulates the hormone insulin, the protein (amino acids, specifically) can be transported at a greater rate into muscle cells for muscle building. Insulin helps transport carbohydrates and amino acids into muscle tissue but excess insulin production can also lead to fat storage. The only time a protein drink should be taken by itself is before bedtime to lower muscle breakdown during sleep.

whey or soy plus whey results in similar increases in lean body mass and does not negatively affect testosterone or estradiol levels in males engaged in a weight-lifting program."

Benefits: Soy protein isolate has a good amount of key amino acids, including glutamine, arginine, and BCAAs, it may boost metabolism by enhancing natural thyroid hormone levels, it contains isoflavones that have been implicated in lowering cholesterol and triglycerides, and it is a lower-cost source of protein.

Downside: Some people complain about the taste of soy products and lower quality soy protein does contain small amounts of phytoestrogens that could boost estrogen levels—not good for men.

Best Uses: Soy is most useful for women, but men can benefit from soy isolates as well. This protein is great for a dieting phase and can be used by anyone to improve general health.

Future Trends

The future of protein products is focused on the key microfractions and components they provide, such as lactoferrin and even colostrum (shown to increase lean muscle mass). More research is being conducted on these microfractions and with advancements in extraction techniques, they may become more cost effective. Some interesting research is focusing on how these microfractions can impact gene expression and overall health. And there will continue to be improvements in taste and consistency of protein powders.

Nutrition Bars

Protein bars are now as prevalent in our society as soda. You can get protein bars at grocery stores, convenience stores, and, of course, health food stores. Protein bars are convenient in that they can be taken with you to work or to the gym. Like meal replacement powders, it is easy to quantify macronutrients in the bar as they are listed on the label. You know how many calories, proteins, carbohydrates, and other nutrients that you are consuming. They can also be cost-effective: a typical protein bar costs around $3, less than a burger and fries. But which protein bars are the best? How can they be beneficial? What do you need to know before purchasing them? Should you buy low-carbohydrate or high-carbohydrate protein bars?

Protein bars usually contain protein, carbohydrates, fat, vitamins and minerals, and additional functional ingredients. High-protein with moderate- to high-carbohydrate bars are best suited for athletes and workout fanatics looking to get quality protein and carbs for increased energy. They are excellent for after a workout to enhance recovery and recuperation and boost carbohydrate storage (glycogen) in muscle tissue. Low-carbohydrate/high-protein bars are good for people looking to maintain lean muscle mass and lose body fat as part of a diet and training program.

The question is "How many carbohydrates are actually in your protein bar?" This question has not only been raised by consumers but also by the U.S. Food and Drug Administration (FDA), which has forced manufacturers to label glycerol and other sugar alcohols (like maltitol) in protein bars as carbohydrates, even though they do not act like carbs in the body—that is they do not cause a significant blood sugar or insulin response after ingestion. That is why the nutritional labels of protein bars have changed and carbohydrate content has shot up drastically with these new regulations. Of course, you'll also see terms like "net impact" carbs or "unavailable" carbs on the label as well with some sort of fancy chart explaining it all. The FDA defines glycerol as a carbohydrate by process of elimination. That is, when a bar is analyzed anything that is not protein, fat, moisture, and ash is considered a carbohydrate. Supplement manufacturers strongly disagree with this, contending that since glycerol is only partially absorbed and does not act like a carbohydrate in the body, it should not be listed as such.

Glycerol (also known as glycerin or glycerine) is a colorless, odorless, sweet-tasting nutrient. It is technically a trihydroxy alcohol found naturally as the backbone of triglycerides in the body, and added to bars to help make them moist and to sweeten them. It does not cause any significant blood sugar response when taken as part of protein bar and seems to be eliminated from the body mostly unused. Glycerol has been shown to enhance athletic performance and cause "hyperhydration" when consumed with water (above and beyond that with water alone). It seems to help keep the body cooler during exercise. Glycerol does contain 4.32 calories per gram, so keep that in mind. However, when glycerol is ingested without water, it can actually cause dehydration. Also, eating too many glycerol-laden protein bars can cause water retention and bloating in some people.

Most nutrition bars contain a significant amount of protein. Some bars may have only one protein source, such as whey protein isolate, but it is better to get a protein blend to utilize all the functional benefits of different proteins and help support lean muscle mass. Look for nutrition bars that contain a blend of whey protein, casein or milk protein isolate, egg albumin, and some soy protein isolate (although bars without soy are fine). Hydrolyzed protein is also another source of protein found frequently in bars because it is inexpensive. This protein is heat treated (and pre-digested) and most of the microfractions are destroyed, thus it is an inferior form.

Another low-quality ingredient popping up in protein bars is hydrolyzed collagen protein, also known as gelatin. This is an incomplete protein that is really cheap. If this protein is in a nutrition bar, I would be cautious about using it, especially if it is one of the main sources of protein. Hydrolyzed collagen does have some benefits in terms of joint and skin health, but not much for building quality muscle. This cheap "pseudo protein" source allows manufacturers to bump up the protein content of bars without adding too much to their costs.

Ask manufacturers of nutrition bars to provide you with an analysis of the proteins in the bar (and for the entire bar, for that matter), which should give you peace of mind about the quality and amount of protein you are getting. Also, bars that contain rolled oats and some granola-type bars are baked and the proteins in them lose the microfractions due to baking. In the basic bar-making process from a quality manufacturer, first the main ingredients (including the proteins) are mixed together (manually or using an industrial-sized mixer) with water, then the mixture is laid evenly on a table and goes through a "cooling" machine. Next, the bar is taken out of the cooling machine and coated with a chocolate coating (enrobed). Finally, the bar sheets are cut and ready to be wrapped. (This is, of course, a simplified version of the process.) This process preserves the microfractions—baking does not.

Protein bars contain carbohydrates as well. Typically, the main sources are sugar alcohols like glycerol (glycerine) and maltitol, especially in "low-carbohydrate" bars. Bars loaded with glycerol and maltitol may cause stomach discomfort in some people, so be sure to drink plenty of water with these protein bars. Corn syrup, high-fructose corn syrup (dextrose), rice syrup, honey (invert sugar), turbinado sugar, sucrose (glucose plus fructose), crisp rice, and fructose are all used as carbohydrate sources in bars.

Fructose is fruit sugar and is added to bars not only to provide a source of carbohydrates but also to sweeten the product (it has a very sweet taste). It is mainly metabolized in the liver and therefore has a lower glycemic index. Consuming higher amounts of fructose can lower metabolic rate and cause fat storage to occur, since the liver can metabolize only a certain amount of fructose. Newer bars have complex carbohydrates such as rolled oats and even brown rice as part of their nutritious blend. An excellent sugar alcohol found in some quality bars is erythritol—this nutrient does not cause a significant blood sugar or insulin response after ingestion and does not seem to cause the stomach discomfort seen with other sugar alcohols. It also helps to sweeten the bar.

Protein bars also contain fat, including partially hydrogenated oils, fractionated vegetable oils, palm kernel oil, and peanut butter. A few bars have added healthy essential fatty acids (EFAs), but it is very difficult to preserve the quality of EFAs due to their sensitivity to light, heat, and oxygen. Most of the fat (especially the saturated fat) found in bars is in the chocolate coating. Saturated fats have been linked to many health problems including cardiovascular disease. Partially hydrogenated oils produce trans fatty acids (along with other altered fats) during the hydrogenation process. They are also very detrimental to health and have been known to increase cholesterol and interfere with the liver's detoxification system. Hydrogenated oils increase the shelf life of products, which is usually nine months to one year for most protein bars. Fractionated oils seem to be better for you. Fractionation is separating an oil into two or more triglycerides based on their chemical properties; it allows weaker oils to be changed into better oils.

Watch out for a high saturated fat content in many nutrition bars. Also, remember that fat provides 9 calories per gram, so high-fat nutrition bar calories can really start adding up. Uncoated bars often have less saturated fat. Some of the better bars on the market are fortified with fat-fighting nutrients like conjugated linoleic acid (CLA), medium-chain triglycerides (MCTs), and sesame oil extract. Look for these ingredients in gram doses in nutrition bars.

Protein bars contain a blend of vitamins and minerals to support overall health and many chemical processes in the body. Vitamins and minerals are usually ancillary items added to bars, but if you have a poor diet, they can help. Whole-food bars like the ZI Diet bar™ and Tri-O-Plex® have set a new standard for whole-grain protein bars. These bars have actual food ingredients like sweet potato, peanut butter, and honey. They taste good and you actually feel like you are eating a food meal. Although, you might want to watch out for the higher fat and calorie content of these bars, depending on your goals. Another great product that is 100 percent vegetarian is Organic Food Bar Inc.'s Vegan Bars™. They contain high-quality ingredients without any "junk."

Usage: As a meal replacement or between-meal protein boost, consume 1–2 bars daily. Drink at least 12–16 ounces of water with each bar. If you have stomach discomfort, eating the bars very slowly and drinking plenty of water can help. When consuming energy bars, take them one hour before a race or an event. Do *not* consume protein bars during exercise as they require water for digestion, which can pull water out of muscle tissues.

LEVEL 2

Essential

Vitamins and Minerals

RECOMMENDED DIETARY INTAKE
FOR ATHLETES (RDIA)

Vitamins and minerals are key nutrients required by the body to allow for optimal function. Deficiencies in certain vitamins and minerals can cause serious disease states and other health problems. The RDA (recommended dietary allowance) is a guideline, designed by nutrition experts for the U.S. government, for the maintenance of good nutrition of practically all healthy people in the United States. It recommends a certain amount of each nutrient, which is basically a bare minimum to help prevent disease.

This is fine for the average person, but what about exercisers and athletes? Active individuals need more of certain nutrients to help them in their training as well as to allow them to prevent a disease condition. So, we'll call this new standard for athletes the Recommended Dietary Intake for Athletes (RDIA). Keep in mind a good multivitamin/multimineral product can provide efficacious amounts of most of these nutrients. Good examples include Opti-Pack from Super Nutrition and Mega Men® from GNC.

VITAMINS

Vitamin A

Vitamin A is also known as retinol and retinal; retinoic acid is a by-product of retinal. "Provitamin A" refers to beta-carotene, which can be converted to retinol in the body. The roles of vitamin A include the visual cycle, cellular differentiation (affects gene expression to control cell development), growth (appears to increase the number of receptors for growth factors), reproductive processes, bone development, and proper immune function. By boosting immune function, vitamin A may create a more favorable environment for muscle growth to occur. Vitamin A works synergistically with zinc and vitamins K and E; a deficiency of these nutrients may impair the function of vitamin A.

RDIA/Dosage: Up to 10,000 IU (international units) in divided doses daily.

Vitamin C

Vitamin C (ascorbic acid) is an essential water-soluble vitamin for any intensely training athlete or dieter. It has several functions in the body, including antioxidant properties, collagen synthesis, immuno-enhancing effects, and decreasing cortisol levels. Vitamin C helps fight free radicals, which are responsible for oxidative damage in the body. Vitamin C has been shown to considerably decrease the duration of cold episodes and the severity of symptoms. If you're sick, you cannot train properly and you may lose hard-earned muscle.

Vitamin C may help reduce unwanted cortisol levels. Cortisol is a catabolic hormone that is secreted in times of stress, such as strenuous weight training. Vitamin C also aids in collagen synthesis. Collagen is a very important substance in the human body: it strengthens the skin, muscles, and bones, and is a primary component of ligaments and tendons. Many studies that document vitamin C's importance for healthy ligaments and tendons, which can be critical for preventing injury and speeding recovery.

Vitamin C also plays a role in fat loss—it is important in the synthesis of the amino acid carnitine. Sufficient carnitine is important in fat metabolism, because carnitine helps transport long-chain fatty acids into the mitochondria for their breakdown to occur. Vitamin C also plays a key role in neurotransmitter synthesis and cholesterol catabolism.

RDIA/Dosage: 1–3 g (grams) in divided doses daily. There isn't a demonstrably superior form of vitamin C on the market, so ascorbic acid is fine. However, Emergen-C™ by Alacer is also an excellent option.

Vitamin D

Vitamin D is associated with skeletal growth and strong bones. Calcitriol is considered the active form of vitamin D and functions like a steroid hormone. It plays a key role in parathyroid hormone, which directs the homeostasis of blood calcium. Parathyroid hormone also stimulates calcium and phosphorus reabsorption in the kidneys. When exposed to sunlight, the body can produce its own vitamin D.

RDIA/Dosage: 400 IU daily.

Vitamin E

Vitamin E includes eight different compounds synthesized by plants. Vitamin E activity is greatest in the alpha-tocopherol form (more specifically, d-alpha-tocopherol). It is a fat-soluble vitamin necessary to maintain membrane integrity in body cells and acts as a powerful antioxidant, preventing the oxidation of unsaturated fatty acids in the cellular membranes. Vitamin E helps fight free radicals: there is an interrelationship between vitamin E and the mineral selenium, as both are tied closely in the function of glutathione peroxidase, a powerful antioxidant. The less muscle breakdown you have by stopping damaging free radicals, the more potential muscle building that can occur. Vitamin E can be regenerated with the help of vitamin C. There was some controversy over a study on vitamin E showing damaging effects, but the study was shown to have many deficiencies. Plus, the overwhelming evidence suggests vitamin E can be beneficial, especially to someone exercising regularly.

RDIA/Dosage: 400–800 IU in divided doses daily. High intakes of vitamin E can interfere with the functions of other fat-soluble vitamins, so I would not recommend taking amounts in excess of 1,200 IU daily. Look for the better absorbed d-alpha-tocopherol form.

Thiamin (Vitamin B_1)

Thiamin is found primarily in the form of thiamin monophosphate in the blood. Thiamin can also be converted to its phosphorylated form, thiamin diphosphate (TDP), in the body. TDP functions as a coenzyme that is necessary for generating ATP (adenosine triphosphate, the primary form of energy used by cells). This is obviously important for promoting muscle function. Vitamin B_1 is also important in nerve conduction and appears to mimic and potentiate the effects of acetylcholine, a neurotransmitter involved in memory.

RDIA/Dosage: 5–10 mg (milligrams) daily. Water-soluble vitamins rarely show any toxicity because excess water-soluble vitamins are excreted in the urine.

Riboflavin (Vitamin B$_2$)

Riboflavin has two coenzyme forms, flavin mononucleotide (FMN) and flavin adenine dinucleotide (FAD), which function in many metabolic reactions in the body. They can act as oxidizing agents and are a part of choline metabolism. Neurotransmitters such as dopamine require FAD for their metabolism: this can stimulate energy levels during exercise, since dopamine can convert to the hormones epinephrine (adrenaline) and norepinephrine (noradrenaline).

RDIA/Dosage: 5–10 mg daily.

Niacin (Vitamin B$_3$)

Niacin, also called nicotinic acid and nicotinamide, can occur as two nucleotides, NAD (nicotinamide adenine dinucleotide) and NADP (nicotinamide adenine dinucleotide phosphate). It can also be formed in the liver from the amino acid tryptophan. NAD helps produce ATP (energy), while NADP is used in a variety of processes, including fatty acid synthesis, cholesterol and steroid hormone synthesis, and oxidation of glutamate. It may also help reduce the oxidized form of vitamin C. Niacin has also been shown to decrease cholesterol levels. Since it acts as a vasodilator, niacin also increases vascularity. It may increase energy during a workout.

RDIA/Dosage: 50–100 mg in divided doses daily. Niacin may cause a flush (redness and vasodilation), especially when taken on an empty stomach. Very high doses of niacin may also be hard on the liver. If you are concerned about these problems, you may want to try the inositol hexonicotinate form, which is easier on the liver. Niacinamide is also a flush-free form of niacin, but a small percentage of the population still seems to have a problem even with this form.

Pantothenic Acid (Vitamin B$_5$)

Pantothenic acid plays an important role in energy storage as well as energy release in the body. It is used, along with cysteine and ATP, to form coenzyme A. As a component of coenzyme A, it is essential for the production of energy from carbohydrates, fat, and protein. Some studies suggest it may also accelerate the healing process, which is important during training.

RDIA/Dosage: 5 mg daily.

Pyridoxine (Vitamin B_6)

The coenzyme form of vitamin B_6 is associated with a vast number of enzymes as part of amino acid metabolism. Vitamin B_6 is also necessary to synthesize heme, the form of iron necessary for optimal blood flow and oxygenation. Niacin synthesis from tryptophan requires pyridoxal phosphate, which is one of the forms of vitamin B_6. It is necessary in glycogen catabolism to "unlock" carbohydrate energy. Vitamin B_6 has also been shown to diminish the actions of glucocorticoid hormones (such as cortisol).

RDIA/Dosage: 5–10 mg daily.

Folic Acid

Folic acid (folate) is necessary in amino acid metabolism and is also required for histidine metabolism (to prevent this amino acid from accumulating in the body). Deficiencies in this vitamin can cause muscle weakness. Ascorbic acid (vitamin C) helps to protect folate from oxidative destruction and there is a synergistic relationship between folate and vitamin B_{12} (cobalamin). This relationship is sometimes called the "methyl-folate trap" because, without vitamin B_{12}, folate is rendered useless in the body.

RDIA/Dosage: 500 mcg (micrograms) daily.

Biotin

Biotin helps many enzymes function in the body, promotes energy metabolism, and is important in the utilization of fats and amino acids. Egg yolks contain a high amount of biotin. Egg whites contain a protein called avidin, which is unstable in heat; it binds to biotin and inhibits its absorption. That is why it is very important to cook egg whites before eating.

RDIA/Dosage: 300–500 mcg daily.

Vitamin B_{12}

Vitamin B_{12} (cobalamin) may boost energy levels and enhance exercise performance. Vitamin B_{12} deficiency can lead to anemia. B_{12} shots are still popular for boosting energy levels.

RDIA/Dosage: 10–15 mcg daily.

Vitamin K

Vitamin K is a fat-soluble vitamin that plays an integral part in blood coagulation. It may also strengthen the bone matrix.
RDIA/Dosage: 50–100 mcg daily.

MINERALS

Calcium

Calcium is the most abundant mineral in the body and about 99 percent of total body calcium is found in the bones and teeth. Calcium has various functions in blood clotting, nerve conduction, muscle contraction, enzyme regulation, and promoting membrane permeability. Only the ionized form of calcium is active and helps perform these functions. Calcium has also been shown to lower blood pressure. Calcium is necessary for the interaction between actin and myosin (muscle proteins), resulting in muscle contraction, so it is vital for exercisers to maintain adequate levels.

You have probably heard since you were a kid that getting enough calcium was essential to grow and have strong bones. This is something well-known among the general population. However, new research has suggested that calcium has benefits beyond just maintaining strong bones. Numerous studies have shown that calcium consumption may lead to significant loss of body fat. One study showed that using calcium supplements (500–2,000 mg daily) actually increased lean body mass and bone mineral density in male athletes. A 2003 study at the University of Tennessee showed that high-calcium diets can increase lipolysis (fat burning) and preserve thermogenesis during calorie restriction. They also mention that low-calcium diets can actually lead to an increase in fat.

It is not exactly known how calcium reduces body fat. One theory is that it helps block digestion and storage of fat. Another theory is that it has positive effects on your hormones to encourage more burning of fat. But contrary to this theory, other research shows that dairy consumption (which is high in calcium) has no impact on fat loss at all. For bone health and just to be safe, try and get 1 gram of calcium daily. The best way to get your calcium is from skim dairy products and calcium citrate supplements.
RDIA/Dosage: 1,000–1,500 mg in divided doses daily.

Phosphorus

Phosphorus is second only to calcium in terms of abundant inorganic elements in the body; approximately 85 percent of phosphorus is found in the skeleton. Most phosphorus is absorbed in the body in its inorganic phosphate form. Phosphorus is extremely important in the metabolism of energy nutrients, contributing to metabolic rate in the form of high-energy phosphate bonds such as ATP (the body's main energy source). Phosphate is also a component of the nucleic acids DNA and RNA. It functions in cell membranes as phospholipids, and is involved in acid-base balance. It may act as a buffer as well, reducing lactic acid buildup. If you can delay or decrease lactic acid buildup, you may be able to train longer and not fatigue as quickly. Studies have shown that supplementing with phosphate increases endurance. Phosphate may also play a role in the formation of phosphocreatine, which can help support the production of ATP.

RDIA/Dosage: 800–1,200 mg daily.

Magnesium

Magnesium ranks fourth in overall mineral abundance in the human body, but intracellularly it is second only to potassium. This mineral is involved in over 300 enzymatic reactions in the body, including glycolysis (the breakdown of carbohydrates into energy), the Krebs cycle, creatine phosphate formation, nucleic acid synthesis, amino acid activation, cardiac and smooth muscle contractability, and, most importantly for bodybuilders, protein synthesis. One study showed that subjects taking magnesium showed increases in absolute strength and lean body mass after seven weeks.

RDIA/Dosage: 500–750 mg daily. Dietary fiber impairs magnesium absorption to a small extent, so I would recommend that you not take magnesium with any fiber source.

Sodium

Sodium is intimately involved with water balance in the body. Sodium constitutes about 93 percent of the cations (positively charged compounds that help regulate pH balance) in the blood. It helps facilitate active transport across all cellular membranes via the sodium-potassium pump. The human body generally requires around 500 mg of sodium daily. However, excess sodium intake can cause water retention in the intercellular space, giving you a bloated appearance. That is why it is important to monitor sodium intake and not consume too much. The major source of sodium in the diet is generally in the form of sodium chloride (table salt).

Dieters need to limit high-sodium foods such as canned meats, processed foods, breads, and certain cereals. It is not advisable to completely restrict sodium intake because the hormone aldosterone may then be released and cause reabsorption of sodium in the kidneys. This will decrease sodium excretion and thus cause you to hold more water. This reabsorption generally takes about twenty-four hours, so I would recommend consuming 1,000 mg of sodium per day the last two weeks before trying to get really lean, and then severely restrict sodium only about eighteen hours before peaking for a competition.

RDIA/Dosage: Try not to exceed 2,500 mg of sodium daily, if you are exercising.

Potassium

Potassium is a macromineral that plays an important role in the contractile functions of smooth, cardiac, and skeletal muscle. It also affects the excitably of nerve tissue and is important in maintaining electrolyte and pH balance. It is part of the sodium-potassium pump that helps transport nutrients across cellular membranes. A potassium-to-sodium ratio of 4:1 should be maintained to optimize bodily functions involving these two nutrients. Potassium can aid in decreasing or lowering muscle cramps, especially with the use of diuretics.

RDIA/Dosage: 2,500–4,000 mg daily (the potassium citrate form if it's from a supplement).

Chloride

Chloride is the most abundant anion (negatively charged particle) in the extracellular fluid (important for pH balance). It is needed for electrolyte balance, because its negative charge neutralizes the positive charge of sodium ions with which it is usually associated. It is also required in the formation of hydrochloric acid, needed for proper digestive function.

RDIA/Dosage: 1,200–1,400 mg daily.

Iron

Iron is a micromineral that is of vital importance to the human body. Iron is an essential component of hemoglobin and myoglobin, parts of the blood that transport oxygen to all the cells of the body and carbon dioxide back to the lungs, where it can be expelled. A deficiency of iron may lead to anemia or a decrease in red blood cells and this can cause lower oxygenation, which may decrease exercise performance as well as lower blood flow into muscle tissue.

There are two forms of iron in food, heme and non-heme iron. Heme iron is mainly found in beef, fish, and poultry; non-heme iron is found in plant foods such as nuts, fruits, vegetables, milk, and eggs. The difference is that non-heme iron is usually bound to components of food and must be hydrolyzed prior to absorption. Heme iron is more easily absorbed than non-heme iron.

RDIA/Dosage: 20–30 mg daily for exercising men and 30–35 mg daily for exercising women. Ascorbic acid has been shown to enhance iron absorption and maintain iron in the appropriate state for enzyme function. Taking 1 g of ascorbic acid (vitamin C) with iron may increase its absorption (especially non-heme iron).

Zinc

Zinc is found in all organs and tissues in the human body. As a component of metalloenzymes, it provides structural integrity to proteins. Zinc is a part of more enzyme systems than the rest of the microminerals combined. It affects many fundamental processes of life—gene expression, cell replication, membrane stabilization—and plays a structural role in hormones such as insulin, testosterone, growth hormone, and estrogen. Zinc deficiency may cause an increased susceptibility to infection and certain skin disorders.

You may have heard the old folktale that eating oysters will put you in a "loving mood" (i.e., high libido), and actually there is science behind this claim. Oysters are an excellent source of highly absorbable zinc, which plays a strong role in maintaining healthy testosterone levels. Several studies have found that zinc consumption is essential for boosting testosterone. One study showed that six months of zinc supplementation actually doubled testosterone levels.

Many studies have shown that zinc supplementation may be a potent immune booster that may reduce the severity and symptoms of colds. Since intense exercise can increase your chances of catching a cold, this immune-enhancing effect is highly important to those who exercise on a regular basis.

RDIA/Dosage: 25–30 mg daily.

Copper

Copper is an enzyme activator in crucial reactions such as the anti-inflamma-tory process and the synthesis of connective tissue. Copper status strongly affects the levels of neuropeptides, enkephalins, and endorphins. This can help support immune function and enhance recovery from workouts.

RDIA/Dosage: 2–4 mg daily. There is an antagonistic relationship be-tween copper and zinc, so do not take copper along with zinc but rather at different times of the day (with food).

Selenium

Selenium is an essential cofactor of glutathione peroxidase, a powerful antioxidant enzyme. It is also involved in pancreatic and immune system function, DNA repair and enzyme activation, and detoxification of heavy metals. Selenium is also necessary for iodine metabolism, which acts in the conversion of T4 to triiodothyronine (T3), the active form of thyroid hor-mone. Selenium may also act as an insulin mimicker, which can help with blood sugar regulation and possibly less fat storage.

RDIA/Dosage: 150–200 mcg daily.

Chromium

Chromium acts to form glucose tolerance factor, which helps insulin bind to its receptor. This action will affect cellular glucose uptake and intracel-lular carbohydrate and lipid (fat) metabolism, which can help improve nutrient uptake into muscle tissue and lower fat storage. Chromium may play a role in fat and cholesterol metabolism by affecting lipoprotein lipase activity. Some studies show it improves blood lipid profiles and causes fat loss.

RDIA/Dosage: 400–800 mcg in divided doses daily.

Iodide

Iodide's main function is in the synthesis of the thyroid hormones by the thy-roid gland. Thyroid hormones stimulate metabolism, oxygen consumption, and heat production. Iodide thus possibly supports fat loss by increasing metabolism.

RDIA/Dosage: 150 mcg daily.

Manganese

Manganese functions both as an enzyme activator and as a constituent of metalloenzymes. A deficiency can cause impaired growth. It increases superoxide dismutase activity (SOD), a powerful antioxidant that may help with the healing and recovery process.

RDIA/Dosage: 15–20 mg daily.

Molybdenum

Molybdenum is a cofactor for four metalloenzymes (xanthine dehydrogenase, aldehyde oxidase, xanthine oxidase, and sulfide oxidase) that function in many different reactions in the human body. This is important for exercisers because these enzymes are involved in muscle recovery and optimal body function.

RDIA/Dosage: 150–200 mcg daily.

Fluorine

The major effects of fluorine or fluoride (which is fluorine bound to either a metal, non-metal, or organic compound) are related to the mineralization of bones and teeth. It may decrease bone resorption, so it is often used to treat osteoporosis. Weak bones can be a problem for exercising individuals and may cause extra pain.

RDIA/Dosage: 2–4 mg daily.

Silicon

Silicon plays a vital role in the formation of bones, connective tissue, and cartilage. It hastens mineralization of bones as well as promotes growth. Silicon has a positive influence on collagen synthesis and is also needed to form glycosaminoglycans, components of the fluid around joints.

RDIA/Dosage: 15–20 mg daily.

Vanadium

Vanadium is both water- and fat-soluble and is present in all healthy tissue. Vanadium may have some insulin-mimicking properties: it can stimulate glucose uptake into cells and enhances glucose metabolism for glycogen synthesis, which can support energy levels and help transport key nutrients into muscle tissue. Foods contain very little vanadium, so supplementation may be necessary.

RDIA/Dosage: 10 mg daily. The vanadate form is up to five times more efficiently absorbed than vanadyl.

Boron

Boron influences the composition, structure, and strength of bones and also plays a role on how certain minerals (such as calcium) are metabolized. This can be a very important factor for athletes.

RDIA/Dosage: 2–3 mg daily.

CMZ™ from VPX Sports is a great mineral product which provides an easy way to supplement mineral intake.

Antioxidants and Free Radicals

Antioxidants aren't very fancy and many athletes and weight trainers don't even take them seriously. When antioxidants are mentioned, everyone looks at their health and protective benefits, but you could also be limiting your muscle-building and fat-burning potential by as much as two-thirds by not taking plenty of antioxidants. That's right, antioxidants can be a powerful tool in your nutritional and fitness arsenal. But why are antioxidants important and how can they help athletes?

What Are Free Radicals?

To understand antioxidants, it is important to review immune function and free radicals (pro-oxidants) and how these damaging compounds work in the body to destroy cells and cause damage to the body. Scientists have found that free radicals carry out much of the destructive work in disease and infection, during stress, and in aging. Free radicals can negatively affect athletic performance by slowing or halting muscle growth and by lowering aerobic capacity. Free radicals are also known to cause defects in the genetic material of the cells (DNA and RNA).

Keep in mind, that some radicals are actually necessary for normal cellular function, but uncontrolled free radical formation can severely threaten the cell. This includes joint tissue and lipid (fat) compounds. Once free radicals start the peroxidation process on lipids, a cascade reaction occurs and cell decomposition or cell death is likely to occur.

Exercise has been shown to increase free radical production, and unless controlled through the use of antioxidants, it can cause a decrease in athletic performance and lean muscle mass. The muscle-destroying activities of free radicals can actually continue many hours and even days after exercise stops. Free radicals may also increase muscle soreness and have been implicated in delayed-onset muscle soreness (DOMS). In fact, at the 2002 National Strength and Conditioning Association national conference, Dr. Malachy McHugh, one of the world's leading researchers on DOMS at the Nicholas Institute of Sports Medicine and Athletic Trauma, stated that there is evidence suggesting that DOMS is caused by free-radical generation and that supplementing with antioxidants may help in this situation. Lowering DOMS can speed up muscle recovery and also reduce that nagging soreness that creeps up about two days after a training session. Antioxidants seem to allow for faster recovery from the inflammatory process.

Normal molecules in the body have two (a paired group) electrons in their outer shell. A molecule with a single electron (unpaired) in its outer shell is called a "free radical." These unstable free radicals occur naturally when oxygen in the bloodstream combines with any of a number of chemicals, including those commonly found in polluted air, in primary or second-hand cigarette smoke, some chemical toxins, in food additives, and in re-heated cooking oil. Think about a time when you cut an apple in half and left it out for a while—it changes to a darker color. What's happening is that it is reacting or oxidizing to the free radicals in the air, thereby disrupting the structural components of the apple.

Antioxidants work by quenching free radicals and converting them into harmless substances. They help stabilize these "unstable" free radicals in different areas of the cell, reducing the pro-oxidant characteristics of these compounds. Your body has a natural antioxidant system of its own, but intense exercise may produce more free radicals than the body can handle on its own without supplementation.

According to Dr. Jan Karlsson, author of *Antioxidants and Exercise,* because most metabolic processes occur in lipid layers and membranes of the cell, protective activity is carried out by the lipid-soluble antioxidant defense. The second line of antioxidant defenses, according to Dr. Karlsson, is in the cytosol in the cell, based on water-soluble antioxidants. So, you have fat-soluble antioxidants and water-soluble antioxidants.

There is a laboratory test that measures antioxidant levels of foods and other nutrients, the Oxygen Radical Absorbance Capacity (ORAC) test. This is the standard by which scientists measure antioxidant activity in foods and supplements. The higher the score using this procedure, the more natural antioxidants in the food. While many whole foods contain high levels of antioxidants, it is also important to take antioxidant supplements along with immune-boosting foods such as wild blueberries, black raspberries, and dark honey.

ANTIOXIDANT FOODS			
Food	ORAC Value (µmoleTE/g)	Food	ORAC Value (µmoleTE/g)
Mango	3	Strawberry	26
Banana	5	Red Raspberry	27
Green grape	6	Plum	28
Kiwi	9	Boysenberry	35
Red grape	11	Blackberry	51
Peach	13	Wild blueberry	61
Apple	14	Pomegranate	105
Raisin	21	Black raspberry	164
Cherry	21	Bee pollen	247
Orange	24		

Values based on limited sample size and fresh weight.
Source: *Health Supplement Retailer* magazine.

Antioxidant Supplements

Now that we know a little about free radicals and immune function, let's review some top antioxidants and immune system–boosting supplements. Although most antioxidants work in much the same way in "disarming" free radicals, it is where they work in the body and how they support immune function that makes them unique.

Vitamin C (Ascorbic Acid)

What is it? Vitamin C is a water-soluble vitamin with proven and potent antioxidant capabilities. It is found in various forms including ascorbic acid, sodium ascorbate, potassium ascorbate, Ester-C, and calcium ascorbate.

What does it do and how does it work? Vitamin C not only acts as a direct antioxidant, but it also supports vitamin E's antioxidant activity by helping regenerate the oxidized form of vitamin E. It is a water-soluble antioxidant that has been shown to lower oxidative stress caused by exercise and to blunt cortisol levels as well. It also seems to decrease post-workout inflammation when taken before a workout.

What does the science say about it? One study showed that taking 2 grams (g) of vitamin C reduced oxidative stress and significantly enhanced recovery. This means you may be able to decrease rest time and get back in the game quicker. Of course, there are numerous studies on its immune boosting effects.

Dosage: Taking 1–3 g daily in divided doses—especially 500 milligrams (mg) to 1 g of vitamin C one hour before training—can be helpful. Emergen-C™ by Alacer is a great vitamin C product.

Vitamin E

What is it? Vitamin E is a fat-soluble antioxidant that works in the lipid parts of the body, such as cell membranes and body fat stores.

What does it do and how does it work? The main function of vitamin E is to maintain membrane integrity in body cells, as it may provide physical stability to membranes. It acts as a powerful antioxidant by preventing the oxidation (peroxidation) of unsaturated fatty acids in the phospholipids of cellular membranes. Vitamin E can be very effective in helping fight free radicals.

What does the science say about it? There are dozens of clinical studies showing the benefits of vitamin E supplementation. A Japanese study published in *Sports Medicine* concluded that supplementation with vitamin E daily should be recommended for all endurance athletes to prevent exercise-induced oxidative damage and also to get the full benefits of exercise.

Dosage: A good dose is 400–800 international units (IU) of vitamin E in divided doses daily, preferably in the natural d-alpha-tocopherol form, which seems to be better absorbed. Taking it with some fat (food or supplement) may aid absorption.

Beta-carotene

What is it? Beta-carotene is a fat-soluble carotenoid that has antioxidant activity and is readily converted to vitamin A in the body (it is a vitamin A precursor).

What does it do and how does it work? Beta-carotene is non-toxic and is only converted to vitamin A in the body as needed. It also may have higher antioxidant activity than pure vitamin A. "Provitamin A" refers to beta-carotene, which can be converted to retinol in the body.

What does the science say about it? Several studies have shown the benefits of combining vitamin C, vitamin E, and beta-carotene in decreasing oxidative stress secondary to exercise in advanced athletes. A study published in the *European Journal of Nutrition* in 2001, and conducted with elite basketball players, showed that this supplement combination enhanced the recovery process and showed signs of reducing muscle breakdown.

Dosage: Good dosages range from 15–30 mg of beta-carotene daily in divided doses (3 mg of beta-carotene supplies around 5,000 IU of vitamin A). Taking it with some fat (food or supplement) may help increase absorption. Be careful about taking very high doses daily as toxicity can be an issue.

Zinc

What is it? The mineral zinc is found in all organs and tissues in the human body.

What does it do and how does it work? As a component of metalloenzymes, zinc provides structural integrity to proteins. Zinc is a part of more enzyme systems than the rest of the microminerals combined. It affects many fundamental processes of life and may also act as an antioxidant, thus supporting immune function.

What does the science say about it? Many studies have shown that zinc supplementation may be a potent immune booster that may reduce the severity and symptoms of colds. Since intense exercise can increase your chances of catching a cold, this immune-enhancing effect is highly important to those who exercise on a regular basis.

Dosage: Typical dosages range from 25–50 mg of zinc daily (preferably in the better absorbed citrate form).

Selenium

What is it? The trace mineral selenium plays a key role in helping to maintain proper levels of the powerful antioxidant enzyme glutathione peroxidase in the bloodstream.

What does it do and how does it work? Selenium is also involved in pancreatic and immune system function, DNA repair, enzyme activation, and detoxification of heavy metals.

What does the science say about it? A large number of studies confirm that selenium plays a preventive and therapeutic role in various diseases. A Canadian review study, published in 2005, discussed how selenium plays a role in many key metabolic functions via its modification of protective selenoproteins.

Dosage: Taking 200 mcg of selenium daily can be beneficial.

Alpha-lipoic Acid

What is it? Also known as lipoic and thioctic acid, alpha-lipoic acid (ALA) is a sulfur-containing antioxidant produced naturally by the body. It can be found in foods such as liver, brewer's yeast, and potatoes.

What does it do and how does it work? Alpha-lipoic acid is both fat- and water-soluble, a powerful antioxidant known as a "universal" antioxidant.

What does the science say about it? Several studies mention that ALA supplementation can reduce oxidative stress and may help maintain structural integrity of cell organelles. So, basically it can help protect cells from damage. One Polish study from 2005 discussed lipoic acid as "a drug of the future" and described its powerful antioxidant effects. What's interesting is that it is actually a prescription medicine in Europe, where it is used to treat diabetic neuropathy.

Dosage: Taking 100 mg of ALA 2–3 times daily can be effective in fighting free radicals. MRM and PrimaForce make some good ALA products.

NAC (N-Acetylcysteine)

What is it? NAC is an amino acid derivative and precursor to glutathione (the body's most powerful water-soluble antioxidant).

What does it do and how does it work? NAC has been shown to increase glutathione levels by up to 500 percent. It can also help support lean body mass and it seems to be a strong free radical scavenger.

What does the science say about it? Several studies show that NAC reduces oxidative stress and can boost immune function. It also seems to enhance liver function. A study conducted at Stanford University, and published in 2000, concluded that NAC supplementation protects against oxidative stress and significantly improves immune function via its enhancement of glutathione.

Dosage: A good dose of N-acetylcysteine is 400 mg taken 2–3 times daily.

Green Tea Extract

What is it? Green tea is a powerful supplement derived from tea leaves that has been widely used for immuno-enhancing effects.

What does it do and how does it work? The major components of interest in green tea extract are polyphenols, including epigallocatechin gallate (EGCG), which seems to provide the strongest antioxidant effects. It helps fight free radicals and support healthy immune function.

What does the science say about it? Most of the research on green tea is focused on its cancer-protective effects. Some research suggests that this potent extract has greater antioxidant protection than vitamins C and E. An Indian study published in 2005 concluded that green tea extract provided greater immunoprotection than vitamin C.

Dosage: Taking 300–400 mg of EGCG daily can be helpful (this equates to about 3–4 cups of green tea). Lean Green™ from PrimaForce is an excellent product.

Proanthocyanidins

What is it? Proanthocyanidins are plant extract antioxidants from grape seed or pine bark. Pycnogenol is another (patented) pine bark extract.

What does it do and how does it work? Proanthocyanidins appear to have a unique ability to increase intracellular vitamin C levels, as well as scavenge free radicals and delay the destruction of connective tissue. The gallic ester form of proanthocyanidins (the most active free radical scavengers) are found only in grape seed extract. The special oligomeric proanthocyanidins (OPCs) seem to be the more potent version in this category and work in both a water- and fat-soluble environment.

What does the science say about it? Several clinical studies show that proanthocyanidins can help protect cells from damage. An Argentinian study published in 2006 states that "procyanidins can exert cytoprotective, anti-inflammatory, and anticarcinogenic actions in the gastrointestinal tract." The research also indicates that they can boost overall health and help fight certain disease conditions.

Dosage: Taking 100 mg daily of an extract containing at least 80 percent proanthocyanidins can be useful. MRM makes a good grape seed extract product.

Goldenseal

What is it? Goldenseal is an immune-boosting herb from the root of *Hydrastis canadensis*.

What does it do and how does it work? Goldenseal supports immune system activity, including the ability to increase the blood supply to the spleen, thus promoting the release of immune-stimulating compounds. In addition, goldenseal helps kill some bacteria and fungi. Its active healing constituent seems to be the alkaloid berberine.

What does the science say about it? Some research suggests that goldenseal boosts immune function and recent research published in the *Journal of Lipid Research* shows that it helps reduce LDL (bad) cholesterol levels. Higher LDL levels have been linked to cardiovascular disease and may have detrimental effects for athletes.

Dosage: It's best to take 400 mg of goldenseal three times a day for a short time, as long-term use can cause the mildly toxic alkaloids in this herb to kill off friendly bacteria in the body.

Echinacea

What is it? Echinacea is an herbal immune system remedy from several species of the purple coneflower (*Echinacea purpurea, E. pallida, E. angustifolia*).

What does it do and how does it work? Although there is some evidence that echinacea may enhance the immune system and reduce some symptoms of a cold, new studies suggest that the remedy may be greatly over-hyped as a means to prevent colds and viral infections. Nonetheless, according to several experts, the latest view on echinacea is that at least 1 g a day may have a subtle effect on reducing the risk of developing a cold.

What does the science say about it? The science is conflicted on whether it works or not, but generally there is validity for its use. For example, an Australian study published in 2005 concludes that echinacea supplementation elicits a positive immune response and increases white cell count. Meanwhile, a German study published in January 2006 states that it is ineffective in an experimental setting.

Dosage: Take 1 g of echinacea a day for three days starting at the onset of a cold.

Astragalus

What is it? Astragalus root is an herb from traditional Chinese medicine used to boost immune function.

What does it do and how does it work? Astragalus can be taken long-term to help build up the immune system, thus boosting its power to prevent and treat viral infections. Traditionally, astragalus has been added to formulations that were aimed at treating weak patients. Astragalus is said to strengthen the spleen, an important organ to immune function.

What does the science say about it? Research suggests it may boost immune function. At least one study shows that astragalus may boost T-cell levels close to normal in some cancer patients, suggesting the use of astragalus with chemotherapy.

Dosage: To benefit from this root, experts recommend taking it in amounts of 6–15 g per day.

Milk Thistle (Silybum marianum)

What is it? Milk thistle is an herb that has been used to support liver function and help with detoxification.

What does it do and how does it work? The main active ingredient seems to be silybin, often gathered with other ingredients as silymarin. It can help with liver damage associated with alcohol consumption, acetaminophen intake, and environmental factors. Having a healthy and optimal functioning liver can also allow for other supplements you take to work more effectively, as most supplements are processed in the liver.

What does the science say about it? Numerous studies show its positive effects as a liver protectant and detoxification agent.

Dosage: Milk thistle is usually standardized for 80 percent silymarin and a dose of 200–300 two times daily can be beneficial.

Two good antioxidant products are Noxidant by SciVation and Super Antioxidants by NOW Foods. Keep in mind that taking too much of any antioxidants may cause a pro-oxidant effect to occur, which would actually create more free radicals. Do not take more than the recommended doses.

Essential Fatty Acids—
Good Fats Can Build
a Better Body

Nutritionists and diet gurus have been indoctrinating us about the evils of dietary fat since the 1970s, so it's difficult to believe that some fats are essential for life. Apparently, the term *fat* is far too simple for the complex substance it represents. Here's why I believe it's in the best interest of everyone—bodybuilders and other athletes as well as everyday folks—to consider supplementing with essential fats: all fats are not created equal.

Essential fatty acids cannot be made by the body and are necessary for life. There are two primary essential fatty acids (EFAs), linoleic acid and linolenic acid. Linoleic acid is an omega-6 fatty acid, while linolenic acid—specifically, alpha-linolenic acid—is an omega-3 fatty acid. Another omega-6 fatty acid, gamma-linoleic acid (GLA), is also important for health and athletic performance. Like water and vitamins and certain amino acids, linoleic and alpha-linolenic acids are required for life. If you don't get them from your diet, your body will deteriorate and you'll die.

A minimal level of EFAs to stave off deficiency hasn't been clearly defined, and there is no RDA (recommended dietary allowance) for either primary essential fatty acid. In the book *Fats That Heal, Fats That Kill* (Alive Books, 1997), author Udo Erasmus suggests a minimum daily intake of 3–6 grams (g) of linoleic acid and 1–3 g of linolenic acid to prevent deficiency. He further suggests that for optimum health, people should take in 3 percent to 6 percent of their calories as linoleic acid and 2 percent as linolenic acid.

EFAs and Prostaglandins

There's a class of "hormones" called prostaglandins in the human body. Certain prostaglandins are beneficial for health and disease prevention, while others are essential to the body's reaction to stress or injury. Prostaglandins (along with immune system substances called leukotrienes) fall into the category of eicosanoids, compounds derived from polyunsaturated fatty acids that can affect cellular activity. There are three classes, or series, of prostaglandins. Series 1 prostaglandins, particularly PGE1, have many beneficial effects for athletes: they appear to have anabolic effects, promote thermogenesis, increase sodium and water clearance by the kidneys, and prevent blood clots. Series 2 prostaglandins have the opposite effects, as they seem to trigger the release of energy substrates by breaking down structural protein, causing salt and water retention and promoting the clotting of blood. Nature always strives to maintain a balance in these processes. In a fight-or-flight situation, your body reacts to ensure your short-term survival: your blood pressure becomes elevated and the energy the body needs becomes available (series 1). When the danger passes, the body seeks to conserve energy (series 2).

One interesting fact is that both series 1 and series 2 prostaglandins are derived from the same precursor, linoleic acid (omega-6), while series 3 prostaglandins are derived from linolenic acid (omega-3). The series 3 prostaglandins are important not for their actions but, rather, for their ability to decrease the rate at which series 2 prostaglandins are formed. So, series 1 prostaglandins promote performance, series 2 prostaglandins disrupt performance, and series 3 prostaglandins block the formation of series 2 prostaglandins. Obviously, athletes want to consume EFAs that help produce series 1 and series 3 prostaglandins.

Prostaglandins are not true hormones. They're paracrine hormones, or in some cases autocrine hormones, which means they are only active in or near the cell where they are generated. True hormones float all through the body to reach distant target organs or tissues. The downside to the local-action-only feature is that prostaglandins aren't orally bioavailable—unless you take them in huge amounts—and can only be administered intravenously. The upside is that you can take the precursors—essential fatty acids—and give your body the building blocks to form prostaglandins naturally.

Health Benefits of EFAs

The positive benefits of EFAs include decreased catabolism and increased growth hormone secretion, improving the action of insulin, enhancing oxygen utilization and energy transformation required for optimal athletic performance, decreasing total serum cholesterol and increasing HDL (good) cholesterol, improving testosterone production, supporting liver function and enhancing immune function, improving the condition of hair and nails, and increasing nitrogen retention. These are all great effects for individuals on a diet and fitness program.

"The latest research for exercising individuals suggests EFAs play a vital role in mediating the excessive inflammation from muscle damage," says Mark Tallon, Ph.D., nutritional biochemist at OxygeniX, a nutrition and supplement research and consulting firm based in London. "Essential fatty acid supplementation may be one method that can dampen down the often excessive inflammation that follows exercise, which over time will allow athletes to recover quicker and adapt faster."

Low-fat diets have been shown to lower testosterone levels. Gamma-linoleic acid may dampen activity of the enzyme 5-alpha reductase, which can lower the conversion of excess testosterone to dihydrotestosterone (DHT), an active form linked to prostate cancer. Eating plenty of EFAs, especially monounsaturated fats, can have a positive impact on testosterone levels. These include natural peanut butter, flaxseed oil, olive oil, and canola oil. Eating fish, including salmon, regularly can also help. One study published in the *Journal of Nutrition* showed that fish oil—containing eicosapentaenoic acid (EPA) and docosahexaenoic acid (DHA)—positively impacted testosterone synthesis. Taking 30–60 g daily of EFAs can be beneficial. In fact, research has indicated that consuming over 20 percent of calories from fats can further enhance testosterone levels. Remember, testosterone is *the* muscle-building hormone.

Taking EFAs

Essential fatty acids have specific chemical structures, including fragile double bonds, that are easily disturbed by heat, pressure, and even light. Oils that contain EFAs must be protected from heat, pressure, and light throughout the pressing, packaging, and shipping processes. Flaxseed oil and evening primrose oil are excellent for fat supplementation. Flaxseed provides a high concentration of omega-3 fatty acids, while evening primrose is a good source of GLA.

Take 20–40 g of essential fatty acids daily (depending on body weight) in divided doses daily. This equates to around 1–3 tablespoons daily, or about 20 percent of body weight in grams. So, if you weigh 200 pounds, you would need 40 g of EFAs daily, which would equate to about 3 tablespoons. Try to consume a 3:1 ratio of omega-3 to omega-6 fatty acids.

Make sure to store EFAs in a cool, dry place (preferably the refrigerator). Look for a blend including flaxseed oil, sunflower oil, fish oils (including EPA and DHA), and olive oil. Special fats like CLA (conjugated linoleic acid) can also help with fat loss. Good EFA blends include Udo's Oil and Total EFA from Health From the Sun.

Amino Acids:
The Forgotten Weapon

Amino acids are the building blocks of protein. There are essential (your body cannot make these) and non-essential (your body can make these endogenously) amino acids. The essential amino acids are tryptophan, lysine, methionine, phenylalanine, threonine, valine, leucine, and isoleucine. The non-essential amino acids include tyrosine, glycine, cysteine, proline, serine, and aspartic acid. They seem fairly ordinary but taking them can have extraordinary effects—that's why I call them "the forgotten weapon" is your quest for fitness success. Let's review some of the top amino acids for exercising individuals.

L-Tyrosine

What is it? The amino acid tyrosine is found in dietary proteins, particularly casein. Many athletes and military personnel have benefited greatly from the use of this underrated supplement.

What does it do and how does it work? L-tyrosine may be useful as a pre-workout energy booster, for mental fatigue or stress, and to increase cognitive function and focus. Tyrosine acts as a direct precursor to the neurotransmitters dopamine, norepinephrine, and epinephrine. It works mainly by stimulating depleted norepinephrine levels in stressed or mentally fatigued individuals. The Naval Aerospace Medical Research Laboratory, in Pensacola, Florida, found that tyrosine played a key role in improving mood and performance in military personnel who are stressed continuously over time. Tyrosine has been called the "focus" supplement because it seems to enhance mental focus and mental clarity. This is especially useful before a workout as mental concentration is essential to sports and exercise performance. Tyrosine has clearly been shown to enhance cognitive performance in stressful situations.

What does the science say about it? A 1994 study showed that tyrosine supplementation improved mental concentration and performance when a stressor was added to the equation. This study also showed that tyrosine had no effects on blood pressure or heart rate. This is good news to those individuals who are sensitive to pre-workout stimulants like caffeine. Other studies have confirmed the positive cognitive effects of tyrosine even during extended sleep loss. One study showed that tyrosine supplementation was beneficial in terms of mental performance after subjects were awake for more than twenty-four hours straight. Anyone who works hard knows the importance of sleep, but when sleep loss does occur, your workouts don't have to suffer if you take L-tyrosine. In fact, during continuous work situations (of more than twelve hours), tyrosine supplementation has been shown to lower fatigue and improve mood.

Tyrosine has been used and extensively researched by the military for years. Research on troops indicates that supplementation with tyrosine significantly lowers stress and fatigue in extremely stressful situations. It is also thought to eliminate any decrease in performance during sustained military operations. It seems to delay mental fatigue and it boosts exercise performance. Since hard weight training is considered a stress to the body, l-tyrosine supplementation may be very useful in improving performance and reducing mental stress. Some recent research confirms the performance-enhancing effects of tyrosine in exercise.

Two good product formulations that contain an effective dosage of Tyrosine are Thermonex EF by BSN and Energize by iSatori Technologies.

Dosage: The recommended dose is 1–3 grams (g) of L-tyrosine, on an empty stomach, one hour before training.

L-Glutamine

What is it? Glutamine is a neutral amino acid and is the most abundant amino acid found in human muscle and blood plasma. Glutamine is sometimes called "conditionally essential" since during times of stress, such as exercise, the body requires more of it to maintain both blood and muscle stores, and higher levels are required for optimal body function and recovery. L-glutamine supplementation can be very beneficial to hard-training athletes.

What does it do and how does it work? Glutamine has a tremendous amount of benefits to exercising individuals and those looking to increase lean muscle mass and decrease body fat. Supplemental glutamine can help promote cell volumization—the drawing of water inside muscle cells—which can help increase muscle "fullness," increase protein synthesis (the making of proteins), and decrease proteolysis (the breakdown of protein). Cellular hydration creates a better environment for muscle growth.

Glutamine has also been shown to aid in recovery and recuperation, help boost immune function by being one of the building blocks for the powerful antioxidant glutathione, possibly cause extra growth hormone release, partially determine the rate of protein turnover in muscles, boost anti-inflammatory cell function, and help increase muscle glycogen deposition through an unknown mechanism.

What does the science say about it? One study actually linked performance decreasing symptoms of the overtraining syndrome in athletes to low levels of L-glutamine in the body. According to some very interesting research out of the Swedish University of Agricultural Sciences, glutamine concentration is 10 percent higher in type II muscle fibers versus type I fibers. Type II muscle fibers have a large disposition for growth and are used mainly in weight training. After exercise, the same researchers showed a 45 percent decrease in glutamine in both fiber types, hence the need for supplementation.

Dosage: Unfortunately, a large majority of ingested free-form L-glutamine does not actually make it into the bloodstream. Up to 85 percent of an oral glutamine load is used by the intestines, liver, and the immune system. This is what many scientists refer to as the "glutamine paradox." Well, with the use of glutamine peptide, this problem may be solved. This form of glutamine is peptide-bonded (a chain of amino acids) to allow for better transport into the bloodstream and muscle tissue where it is needed. Wheat protein hydrolysate is a common source for glutamine peptide.

A good dose is 5–10 g of glutamine or glutamine peptide consumed right after a workout. The best time to take a glutamine supplement is right after a hard exercise session, since glutamine stores in muscle can be depleted up to 40 percent after exhaustive exercise. Then, take 5 g 1-1/2 hours after training. Another 5 g before bedtime can also be beneficial during a really hard training cycle or competition.

Branched-Chain Amino Acids (BCAAs)

What are they? Branched-chain amino acids (BCAAs) include the essential amino acids leucine, isoleucine, and valine. They are very popular among athletes and there is some research validating their use.

What do they do and how do they work? These three key amino acids are extremely important to consume, especially when you are dieting and exercising (BCAAs are even more important when exercising in the heat). During exercise, your body uses a mix of glucose, fats, and even protein as a fuel source. When you diet and your carbohydrate intake is lower than normal, the percentage of protein your body uses for fuel (specifically, the BCAAs) dramatically increases. The body will pull the needed amino acids from the continuously circulating pool of amino acids in your bloodstream. And if not replenished from an outside source—specific amino acid ingestion in the form of BCAAs—your body will break down other areas of your body in order to supply this pool.

What does the science say about them? Studies have shown that subjects who consume an effective dose of BCAAs while dieting have greater levels of lean muscle mass retention than controls who ingest a placebo (the control subjects typically *lose* muscle during the same dieting period). Results from one study concluded that the subjects consuming a high-protein diet including branched-chain amino acid supplements lost the greatest amount of body fat. Even more compelling is that the group supplementing with BCAAs lost the greatest amount of fat from the abdominal and thigh regions, two areas of concern for many men and women. BCAAs (particularly leucine) are also being looked at in the area of genetic modification and expression, a very interesting topic for cutting-edge research.

Dosage: It is important to take 1 gram doses of each of the BCAAs before, during, and after exercise to maximize a workout program.

L-Arginine

What is it? L-arginine is a non-essential amino acid that can have many positive effects in exercising individuals. It is considered "conditionally essential" because even though it is synthesized by the body, it is not made in high enough amounts to support growth functions or to meet the needs of individuals under times of stress (such as sports competition or hard weight training).

What does it do and how does it work? Arginine has many beneficial effects for cardiovascular health. It may help lower cholesterol and it seems to boost immune function and wound healing as well. It is also a precursor to natural creatine production in the body (creatine is made in the body from the amino acids glycine, arginine, and methionine). So, it can have a "creatine sparing" effect, which may be beneficial for increasing strength. It may help improve exercise performance, support protein synthesis, and even help replenish glycogen (stored carbohydrate) stores post-workout.

What does the science say about it? A 2002 study published in the *International Journal of Sports Medicine* showed that arginine supplementation helped reduce lactate and ammonia build-up during exercise. This can help delay muscle fatigue, which is good news for athletes. Some research shows it improves insulin sensitivity, thereby allowing carbohydrates to be used more effectively by the body. Its main mechanism of action is boosting nitric oxide (NO) production. NO is the muscle cells' "signaling molecule"— boosting nitric oxide in muscle tissue can have many anabolic effects, including increased nutrient transport and vasodilation (increased blood flow, which could lead to better muscle pumps). Arginine boosts NO by stimulating nitric oxide synthase, the enzyme that makes NO.

L-arginine has equivocal evidence that it can boost growth hormone (GH) levels. Some studies show little effect of L-arginine as a GH booster, while other studies, such as one published in *Medicine and Science in Sports and Exercise* in 1999, shows good effect. A published study conducted at Sinai Hospital, in Baltimore, showed that two weeks of arginine supplementation in healthy, older individuals increased serum IGF-1 (insulin-like growth factor 1) levels and created a positive nitrogen balance (producing a more anabolic state for growth). Growth hormone seems to have many of its positive muscle-building effects due to its conversion into IGF-1 in the liver.

Dosage: Hard-training athletes can certainly benefit from 5–10 g of L-arginine daily. Important times to consume L-arginine are 45 minutes before and right after a workout session to enhance the recovery process (3–5 g taken at both these times should help). However, caution is advised because, in some people, gram doses of arginine may cause stomach discomfort. Arginine has a good safety record even at high doses of 20+ g consumed daily. L-arginine can be found in tablet, capsule and powder form. The powder form may be the most convenient way to take good amounts of arginine unless you prefer swallowing lots of pills.

Some recommended amino acid–based combination products include: BCAA 5000 Powder from Optimum Nutrition, Recoverzene from ASR, NO Shotgun from VPX Sports, GlutaLean from Labrada, Energize by iSatori Technologies, Nitrix from BSN, Muscle Armor from EAS, and Aminovol from NxCare.

LEVEL 3

Performance

Fat Loss

Fat burning is a very sophisticated and detailed biochemical process. Fat contains 9 calories per gram, which makes it the most energy-dense macronutrient. Fatty acids are stored as triglycerides in adipose (fat) tissue. Each triglyceride molecule consists of three fatty acids and one glycerol unit. Burning 1 gram (g) of fat for fuel provides more energy than burning a gram of carbohydrate.

Obesity or greater fat storage usually results from a continuous imbalance between energy intake and energy expenditure. The key to fat loss is lowering energy intake and/or increasing energy expenditure (possibly through thermogenesis) Fats are oxidized (burned) to provide energy through a process called beta-oxidation (lipolysis). So, fat burning can impact overall body heat expenditure.

Thermogenic Supplements

The idea behind thermogenic nutrients is to boost body metabolism so that you can naturally burn more calories. This category is booming since it seems like everyone is looking to shed some extra pounds and get lean abs. Stimulant fat burners are increasingly popular, so it's time to investigate some of these thermogenic weight-loss ingredients and shed some light on this supplement category.

Caffeine

What is it? Caffeine belongs to a group of chemicals called xanthines (more specifically, it's a trimethylxanthine). It exerts many of its useful effects due

73

to its chemical structure—caffeine is considered by many to be a drug. The herbal versions of caffeine include guarana and kola nut.

What does it do and how does it work? Caffeine works through several mechanisms of action, including promoting the release of stored fat to be used as energy, more release of calcium from the sarcoplasmic reticulum in muscle tissue (thereby leading to greater muscle contraction and force production), antagonism of the adenosine receptors mainly in the central nervous system (which can help enhance focus and mental function), and inhibition of phosphodiesterases leading to an increase level of cyclic AMP in muscle tissue (creating a more favorable intracellular environment in active muscle). Caffeine also spares glycogen (carbohydrate stores in muscle cells and the liver) leading to an increased rate of fat oxidation, which could explain why caffeine delays time to exhaustion during aerobic exercise.

Caffeine has some diuretic properties that can aid in decreasing water retention in the body, although it does not seem to act as a diuretic during exercise. Nevertheless, it is important to consume plenty of water when taking in caffeine. Another thing to look out for is caffeine's effects on blood sugar. Although not clear from the research, it may decrease insulin sensitivity, so diabetics need to be careful. Regularly consuming high amounts of caffeine may also adversely affect blood pressure. Moderation is the key.

What does the science say about it? Caffeine is one of the best-researched ergogenic (capable of enhancing physical performance) aids available. It has been shown in several studies to promote fat oxidation and both weight loss and fat loss in exercising individuals. Many studies show that caffeine enhances both short-term and long-term endurance. Caffeine seems to delay fatigue (prolongs time to exhaustion), so aerobic workouts can go on longer and stronger. It has been shown to be effective in increasing speed in simulated race conditions. A 1998 study published in the *International Journal of Sports Medicine* found that caffeine was an effective ergogenic aid for short-term, maximal running performance. Even though there are far fewer studies with caffeine and resistance training (weight lifting), some evidence suggests that caffeine can increase power generated in repeated muscle contractions and enhance endurance at submaximal tension.

A combination of *guarana* and *Yerba maté* (and *Damiana* leaf), containing a good dose of caffeine, was shown in a study published in the *Journal of Human Nutrition and Dietetics* to significantly enhance weight loss after just 45 days of use, and they kept their weight off for a full year after the study.

Dosage: A regular cup of coffee has about 100 milligrams (mg) of caffeine but some research shows that coffee is not as effective in maximizing the

Caffeine Precautions and Side Effects

- Calcium Absorption and Bone Health—There is some link between caffeine consumption and bone health, especially in women. However, if adequate amounts of calcium are being consumed, caffeine does not pose a problem at all.

- Blood Pressure—Research shows that moderate caffeine consumption daily does not elevate blood pressure in healthy individuals, but higher doses of caffeine (5 cups of coffee daily) have been linked to high blood pressure. Moderation is the key. If you have pre-existing high blood pressure, then caffeine should be avoided.

- Homocysteine Levels—Heavy coffee drinking raises plasma homocysteine levels. Since an elevated level of total homocysteine is considered to be a risk factor for cardiovascular disease, it is a good idea not to overdo it with caffeine on a regular basis.

- Stomach Discomfort—No research suggests this clearly, but some people who take higher doses of caffeine complain of mild stomach distress. If this is a problem, then taking caffeine with food may help. This may also subside after several days of caffeine use.

- Jitteriness and Nervousness—Since caffeine is considered a stimulant, some people may experience these effects. Lowering the caffeine dose initially may help and some of these symptoms may subside after caffeine tolerance is reached.

Pregnant and nursing women should be aware that some evidence suggests that taking more than 300 mg of caffeine daily may increase the risk of miscarriage and a low–birth weight baby. Caffeine crosses the placenta and affects the unborn baby and it is also transferred into breast milk. It's definitely a good idea to avoid caffeine while pregnant or nursing.

benefits of caffeine as is pure caffeine (in pill, powder, or liquid form). A good dose is 100–300 mg consumed forty-five minutes before a workout, especially cardiovascular exercise. As mentioned earlier, the best form is pure caffeine, but guarana and kola nut also contain caffeine.

Cayenne Pepper

What is it? Cayenne pepper contains capsaicin, which is the compound that produces the "hot" in hot peppers. Cayenne peppers have been used for centuries to relieve many ailments, including digestive problems and pain.

What does it do and how does it work? Cayenne has unique metabolic and thermogenic properties based on its capsaicin (the active ingredient) content. Cayenne pepper has been noted for hundreds of years to increase perspiration and influence body temperature. Its effects on thermogenesis are mainly attributed to capsaicin's activation of the sympathetic nervous system (stimulation of the hormones epinephrine and norepinephrine). This results in enhanced energy metabolism, more calories being used, and a feeling of warmth.

What does the science say about it? According to research, cayenne pepper can help decrease appetite and lowers food intake. Newer research from Australia suggests that it can help stabilize insulin levels after a meal—this may mean less fat storage and better energy levels.

Dosage: When looking for a cayenne pepper product, make sure it contains a standardized amount of capsaicin. A good dose is 30 mg three times daily. (I sprinkle cayenne pepper on each of my food meals to really fire things up.)

Evodiamine

What is it? Evodiamine is a major alkaloid found in the *Evodia* fruit family, commonly called *Evodia rutaecarpa* or *Evodiae fructus*. It is reported to have many characteristics of cayenne, including thermogenesis and analgesic (pain relief) use, without the same hot peppery effect. *Evodia* fruit is commonly used in China for its positive effects on digestive disturbances.

What does it do and how does it work? Evodiamine has been shown to have promise in increasing metabolism and reducing fat storage. There is also evidence that points to appetite suppression by way of increasing cholecystokinin (CCK), a hormone responsible for sending a signal to the brain to stop eating, and delayed gastric emptying.

What does the science say about it? Despite a lack of human clinical trials using evodiamine, there are still promising results when it comes to fat loss. In a 2001 research article in *Planta Medica*, rats given evodiamine showed significant fat loss compared to a control group. An interesting finding of the study was that evodiamine could induce heat loss at the same time as a heat production increase. This indicates less fat storage and weight gain from food intake. From this, the researchers concluded that there was a more efficient use of food energy when evodiamine was used. In the same study, there was evidence that evodiamine may effectively stimulate brown adipose tissue thermogenesis, which points to a heightened fat loss effect. So, similar to it's capsaicin counterpart, evodiamine has effective metabolism boosting and fat loss properties, without the fiery kick.

Dosage: Look for evodiamine standardized to at least 10 percent. An effective amount is 40 mg taken in two divided doses daily.

Green Tea Extract

What is it? Green tea is gulped daily by people of many cultures around the world. The major components of interest in green tea extract are the polyphenols, including epigallocatechin gallate (EGCG).

What does it do and how does it work? Green tea seems to boost metabolism, help with weight loss, support healthy immune function, and improve overall health. It's the phytochemicals (plant chemicals) in green tea extract, including EGCG, that are responsible for its many positive effects. Green tea extract may increase fat oxidation and even stimulate brown adipose tissue thermogenesis (special fat cells can that actually work for you to speed up metabolism)—good news for anyone looking to lose body fat.

What does the science say about it? Most of the research on green tea has focused on its cancer-protective effects. Some research suggests that this potent extract has greater antioxidant protection than vitamins C and E. But what many people don't know is that it may have great potential as a fat burner. A 1999 study published in the *American Journal of Clinical Nutrition* showed that green tea extract increased 24-hour energy expendi-

A QUICK GUIDE TO THERMOGENIC SUPPLEMENTS

Caffeine

ACTIVE INGREDIENTS: A compound chemically referred to as a trimethyl-xanthine. The benefits of caffeine are due to its chemical structure. Effective herbal caffeine sources include guarana and kola nut.

ACTIONS: Several studies have indicated that caffeine may accelerate fat loss and enhance muscle contraction and force production. Benefits also include an increase in focus and enhanced endurance.

RECOMMENDED DOSE: 100–300mg of pure caffeine in pill, powder, or fat-loss formula form forty-five minutes before exercise.

Cayenne Pepper

ACTIVE INGREDIENTS: Capsaicin is the main constituent and is the compound responsible for the "hot" flavor. Capsaicin has been used for centuries to enhance digestion, relieve pain, and increase perspiration.

ACTIONS: Cayenne has been shown to increase thermogenesis (fat burning) by activating the sympathetic nervous system. Research also indicates that it may curb appetite and stabilize insulin levels, leading to less fat storage.

RECOMMENDED DOSE: 30 mg standardized for capsaicin, three times daily. May be taken with meals.

Evodiamine

ACTIVE INGREDIENTS: Evodiamine is a standardized alkaloid extract from the *Evodia* fruit.

ACTIONS: Evodiamine has promising evidence for fat loss and inhibiting fat gain due to enhanced food energy usage. There is also promise regarding appetite suppression.

RECOMMENDED DOSE: 40 mg standardized for 10 percent evodiamine, two times daily.

Green Tea Extract

ACTIVE INGREDIENTS: Its main components are polyphenols, including epigallocatechin gallate (EGCG), and some caffeine.

ACTIONS: A host of benefits, including increased thermogenesis and fat oxidation, healthy immune function, and improvement in overall health.

RECOMMENDED DOSE: 400–700 mg daily, in two divided doses. Look for standardized extract of at least 40 percent EGCG.

Citrus Aurantium (bitter orange, zhi shi)

ACTIVE INGREDIENTS: Active components include synephrine (calmer chemical cousin of ephedrine) as well as octopamine and tyramine.

ACTIONS: Synephrine shows promising results for fat loss. Although less stimulating than ephedrine, it shows similar effects on increasing metabolism.

RECOMMENDED DOSE: 20–40 mg of synephrine in divided daily doses. One serving should be taken one hour prior to exercise.

---

ture and fat oxidation in humans. This may be due to its caffeine content, since caffeine has some of these properties, but the authors of this study concluded that "green tea extract has thermogenic properties and promotes fat oxidation beyond that explained by its caffeine content per se. Green tea extract may play a role in the control of body composition via sympathetic activation of thermogenesis, fat oxidation, or both." Its effectiveness is most likely linked to the EGCG content.

Another study showed the synergy of green tea's catechin polyphenol and caffeine content in stimulating brown adipose tissue thermogenesis. This means that green tea extract may be a valuable tool in assisting in the management of obesity. Another study published in the *American Journal of Clinical Nutrition* showed that a dose of approximately 600 mg per day of a green tea extract for twelve weeks significantly reduced body weight.

Dosage: A good dose of green tea extract is 400–700 mg in two divided doses daily. Look for a standardized extract containing at least 40 percent EGCG. The pill form is the way to go as you would have to drink four to six cups of tea to get the same amounts of the active ingredients.

Citrus Aurantium

What is it? *Citrus aurantium* (bitter orange or zhi shi) is an herb that contains the active ingredient synephrine, along with other potent compounds like octopamine and tyramine. Synephrine is touted as an ephedra alternative, since ephedra was banned by the FDA in April 2004.

What does it do and how does it work? Synephrine is ephedrine's calmer chemical cousin, which means it still has thermogenic/fat-burning effects while being less stimulating to the central nervous system. However, its lipolytic effects in fat cells may only be effective at high doses. Synephrine may enhance metabolism and increase blood pressure (temporarily, at least).

What does the science say about it? A 1999 study in *Current Therapeutic Research* showed that a combination of *Citrus aurantium* extract, caffeine, and St. John's wort caused significant body fat loss in overweight healthy adults (synephrine was the key). Other research has looked at the thermogenic properties of compounds found in *Citrus aurantium,* including synephrine and octopamine, and the results look very promising. And a review article in *Obesity Review Journal* in 2006 stated that synephrine showed some promising effects for fat loss.

Dosage: Typical doses range from 20–50 mg of synephrine in divided doses daily, preferably taking one dose an hour before exercise. Taking it too close to bedtime may interfere with sleep.

Quality thermogenic products that contain many of these ingredients include Lean System 7 and MX-LS7 from iSatori Technologies, Methyl Ripped from NxLabs, Lipo-6 from Nutrex, Hydroxycut® from MuscleTech™, and Redline from VPX Sports. For an additional boost, take the recommended dose (with plenty of water, of course) forty-five minutes before training, especially before a cardiovascular workout.

Please be advised that thermogenics are very powerful products that are for healthy, exercising individuals. If you have any medical conditions (especially high blood pressure, cardiovascular problems, or thyroid issues) or are taking medications, it is vital to consult your physician before taking any of these potent nutrients.

Non-Stimulant Fat-Loss Agents

Non-stimulant fat-loss agents have saved the day for many thermophobic people. There was definitely a need for these types of products as many people were not only getting "burned out" using thermogenic supplements but others were actually very sensitive to the ingredients, such as caffeine, in stimulant fat burners. Non-stimulant fat burners can still be quite effective in terms of fat loss. For those people that do not have a problem using stimulant supplements, these non-stimulant products can be combined with them to further promote fat burning. However, watch out for doubling up of ingredients.

Bioperine®

What is it? Bioperine is derived from black pepper, a spice most households have in the kitchen cupboard. A compound called piperine, the active ingredient, comes from an extract of the small pepper berry.

What does it do and how does it work? Piperine has been shown to significantly enhance the absorption of various supplemented nutrients, while generating an increase in metabolic action to help support fat loss. The higher the metabolic rate, the more heat energy is produced by the body, therefore, enhancing the fat-burning process.

What does the science say about it? Clinical trials showed that Bioperine is a natural thermonutrient and bioavailability enhancer. There is a lot more information on this at www.bioperine.com.

Dosage: A good dose of Bioperine is 5 mg taken 1–3 times daily, preferably with other fat-loss nutrients in a formula.

Conjugated Linoleic Acid (CLA)

What is it? Conjugated linoleic acid (CLA) has been shown in many recent studies to have profound fat-loss effects in humans. This advanced form of an essential fatty acid can help reduce body fat while dieting. It is naturally found in beef and dairy products, but supplementation is the only way to get efficacious doses.

What does it do and how does it work? CLA can help increase lean body mass and it has other health benefits in the body including acting as an antioxidant. Researchers have proposed several mechanisms by which CLA works. It apparently interferes with a substance in the body called lipoprotein lipase that helps your body store fat and CLA also helps your body use its existing fat for energy. So, you prevent fat storage while burning the fat you have.

What does the science say about it? Recent long-term research on Cognis' Tonalin® CLA showed that it caused a significant decrease in body fat while increasing lean body mass over a one-year study. CLA supplementation for a year caused a 9 percent reduction in body fat and a 2 percent increase in lean muscle mass. Another study conducted at Maastricht University in the Netherlands showed that CLA may support the regaining of fat-free mass after weight loss. This 2003 study, published in the *International Journal of Obesity and Related Metabolic Disorders,* also showed that CLA supplementation at a dose of either 1.8 g or 3.6 g daily caused an increase in resting metabolic rate.

A 2003 study published in the *Journal of Nutrition* showed that CLA had positive effects on fasting blood sugar levels and may have some uses for treating type II diabetes. The researchers even theorized that CLA may have an effect on appetite due to its modification of the hormone leptin.

Not all the research with CLA in humans is positive, however. One study conducted at the University of Memphis concluded that CLA supplementation did not affect body fat, lean body mass, or strength. This was a relatively short-term study (28 days). One interesting thing to note is that CLA has many patents on it for many functions, including lean muscle gain, altering body fat levels, and even treating diabetes.

Dosage: Effective doses of CLA range from 1.4–4.2 g daily. There are two main forms of CLA (cis 9,11 trans or cis 10,12 trans) and using a mixture of the two seems to be the most effective. A great CLA-based product is Abgone™ from Biotech Research.

Coleus Forskohlii

What is it? *Coleus forskohlii* (active ingredient, forskolin) is a "power" herb that may be a good supplement for fitness enthusiasts.

What does it do and how does it work? *Coleus forskohlii* increases the amount of cyclic AMP (adenosine monophosphate) in cells by activating an enzyme called adenylate cyclase. Why is it important to increase cAMP levels? Well, there are several benefits of this to athletes, including relaxation of the arteries and smooth muscles, lowering blood pressure, enhanced insulin secretion (which can help drive carbohydrates and protein into muscle cells for energy and recovery), increased thyroid hormone function (which can help enhance metabolic rate), and significantly increased lipolysis (fat burning). Forskolin also seems to benefit other cellular enzymes as well.

What does the science say about it? Forskolin has been shown not only to enhance lipolysis but also to inhibit fat storage. It is patented by the Sabinsa Corporation for stimulating lean body mass (the more lean muscle mass you have, the more calories you will burn at rest, hence more fat loss). A 2002 study showed that forskolin (ForsLean®) helped mitigate weight gain and was proven to be very safe. New research on ForsLean is showing some promising results in terms of natural testosterone enhancement.

Dosage: A good dose is 100 mg of *Coleus forskohlii* standardized to 20 percent forskolin. Taking 25–60 mg of forskolin daily in divided doses can be beneficial.

Guggulsterones

What is it? Guggulipid (also known as guggulsterones) has been around for hundreds of years in Ayurvedic medicine, a naturalistic approach to medicine that has been practiced in India for centuries. It is found as a component of the plant *Commiphora mukul*.

What does it do and how does it work? To begin the discussion about guggulipid, we must first talk about thyroid hormone. Thyroid hormones maintain metabolic stability by regulating oxygen requirements, body weight, and intermediary metabolism. Thyroid hormones also exert effects on thermogenesis and temperature regulation. They can enhance lipolysis (fat burning) in adipose (fat) tissue. The two main thyroid hormones are T4 (thyroxine) and T3 (triiodothyronine). T4 is inactive thyroid hormone while T3 is active thyroid, but T4 can convert into T3 in the liver. Guggulsterones help normalize and optimize proper thyroid hormone function by enhancing the uptake of iodine.

What does the science say about it? There have been several research studies done on this herb showing very positive benefits. A 1989 study in the *Journal of Association of Physicians in India* showed that guggulipid had a very strong effect on decreasing triglycerides (fats) as well as LDL (bad) cholesterol levels while increasing HDL (good) cholesterol levels in human subjects. It has these functional effects because it may cause an increase in thyroid hormone levels (both T4 and T3). There are several other studies that have shown similar effects of guggulipid as a fat-reducing compound. A 2004 study published in *Atherosclerosis* concluded that "the combination of antioxidant and lipid-lowering (fat reducing) properties of *C. mukul* and guggulsterone makes them especially beneficial against atherogenesis."

Many people following a diet and training program over a fairly long period of time complain that they just cannot lose that last bit of fat no matter what they do. Well, thyroid hormones may play a key role in this process. Your body adapts to any diet program involving a caloric deficit by reducing thyroid hormone output. By taking guggul, thyroid hormones can be normalized and you can continue burning fat. This natural compound has also been shown to be very safe and completely nontoxic. However, one study published in the *Journal of the American Medical Association* showed that it slightly raised levels of the LDL cholesterol, but the study was not conclusive.

Dosage: When choosing a guggulipid product, make sure it is a standardized guggulsterone of type E and Z from the plant *Commiphora mukul*. A good dose is 25 mg of active guggulsterones taken three times daily. One dose with plenty of water 30 minutes before cardiovascular exercise can be helpful.

Hydroxycitric Acid (HCA)

What is it? Hydroxycitric acid (HCA) or hydroxycitrate is the main acid derived from the fruit of the *Garcinia cambogia* tree, found mainly in Southeast Asia. This is certainly not a new ingredient; in fact, it has been studied quite extensively for years.

What does it do and how does it work? HCA acts as an appetite suppressant through enhancement of serotonin levels (by stimulating its release and inhibiting its re-uptake). Increasing serotonin levels has been shown to decrease food intake, enhance mood, and lower weight gain. Controlling food intake is a key determining factor to losing fat. HCA is thought to help with weight loss by inhibiting an enzyme called ATP citrate lyase, which helps convert excess carbohydrates to fat in the liver. However, there is some question about whether or not this enzyme is very active in humans.

What does the science say about it? Animal studies have been fairly consistent in showing the usefulness of this ingredient, but that doesn't mean it necessarily works for humans looking to lose weight. Human studies with HCA have been equivocal: several studies show no effect of HCA on weight loss while other studies show good effects from this ingredient. One fairly large, well-controlled study published in the *Journal of the American Medical Association* in 1998 concluded that *Garcinia cambogia* failed to produce significant weight loss and fat mass loss. This study used a low dose of 1,500 mg daily of HCA and the subjects in the study were on a low-calorie diet. These may be some reasons why the HCA did not produce significant results. Higher doses seem to be necessary to have an effect on weight/fat loss. Other studies on HCA using a similar low dose have shown no significant effect as well.

However, a study at Georgetown University Medical Center showed much better results with HCA supplementation. Individuals using HCA lost a significant amount of weight, lowered their total cholesterol (and raised their HDL cholesterol), and experienced appetite suppression through increased serotonin levels after eight weeks of supplementation. The HCA used in this study was a more potent extract called Super CitriMax® from Interhealth. The dosage and timing of ingestion is the key with HCA supplementation. This study used 2,800 mg of HCA daily, given thirty minutes before meals in three divided doses. On the contrary, another recent study suggests lower doses may be useful for appetite suppression. This study from the Netherlands showed that 300 mg HCA taken three times daily reduced energy intake while sustaining satiety.

Dosage: HCA should be taken thirty minutes before meals three times daily for at least four weeks. An efficacious dose for weight loss is 2,500 to 3,000 mg daily of active HCA (after standardization from *Garcinia cambogia*) in divided doses. For appetite suppression, lower doses may be helpful. HCA seems to be very safe, with no side effects reported in the majority of the human studies. Although, not highly rated, it may be effective nonetheless. Good HCA supplements include CitriMax from Optibolic (available at GNC) and Hydroxycut® from Muscletech™.

7-Keto DHEA

What is it? 7-Keto DHEA is a metabolite of DHEA (dehydroepiandrosterone), a natural hormone produced by the adrenal glands.

What does it do and how does it work? According to the research, 7-Keto DHEA may boost levels of the thyroid hormone T3. This can lead to an increased metabolism and greater fat burning. Because 7-Keto DHEA does not convert into the sex steroids (testosterone and estrogens), it can have many of the benefits of DHEA, such as increased energy, sex drive, and even fat loss, without any unwanted side effects.

What does the science say about it? Several studies show that this patented compound can have powerful fat-burning effects in healthy individuals. One study published in *Current Therapeutic Research* in 2000 showed that 7-Keto DHEA caused three times more fat loss versus a placebo.

Dosage: A typical dose of 7-Keto DHEA is 100 mg taken 1–2 times daily. A good source of 7-keto DHEA is Lean System 7® by iSatori Technologies, or MX-LS7™.

L-Carnitine

What is it? The amino acid L-carnitine is a vitamin-like compound that may enhance fat utilization when taken prior to exercise, although research on this nutrient has been equivocal (some positive and some negative).

What does it do and how does it work? L-carnitine works by promoting the transport and metabolism of long-chain fatty acids into the mitochondria of cells to be burned as fuel (beta oxidation) and used for energy. It is a naturally occurring compound found in meats and dairy products. That is why vegetarians may benefit most from supplementation. L-carnitine has been shown to have some cardioprotective effects as well.

What does the science say about it? Some research suggests that L-carnitine may enhance endurance, since fat is the major metabolic fuel for long-term aerobic exercise. In terms of weight loss, a fairly high dose (2 g twice daily) was shown to have no effect on fat loss when combined with light exercise in overweight women. The problem may be getting carnitine into muscle tissue.

This supplement may have some uses but it certainly has not lived up to its hype. Most products on the market contain low doses of carnitine just to claim that they have it. There is some new research that shows that L-carnitine L-tartrate (a special form) can actually assist significantly in recovery from hard training and this may prove to be one of its best uses.

Dosage: I wouldn't recommend L-carnitine for fat loss until more comprehensive research is done, but for exercise recovery, taking 1–2 g one hour before training can be helpful. Liquid L-carnitine supplements may be better absorbed. Watch out for low milligram doses in products. Optimum Nutrition makes a great L-carnitine L-tartrate product.

Phosphates

What is it? Phosphates are mineral compounds that contain phosphorus and may help boost metabolism and possibly exercise performance.

What does it do and how does it work? Potassium phosphate may enhance recovery after exercise. Phosphates may also delay fatigue by buffering lactic acid and they can help store creatine better in muscle cells (since creatine is stored as creatine phosphate). This can help support greater energy production and resynthesis in the muscle tissue, which could lead to exercise performance enhancement.

What does the science say about it? According to a 1996 study published in the *Journal of Physiology and Pharmacology,* a combination of calcium, potassium, and sodium phosphates were shown to increase resting metabolic rate in overweight women who were on a low-calorie diet. The authors of this study concluded that phosphates may play a role in the peripheral metabolism of thyroid hormones, specifically by preventing a decrease in T3 output. Thus, metabolism and fat burning may be increased. Another study published in 1993 showed that calcium and potassium phosphate supplementation is useful in increasing metabolic rate and helping with fat loss.

Dosage: A good dose is 1 g of phosphates taken one hour prior to exercise. Some people may experience stomach discomfort with this dose so a lower dose may be used to allow the body to adapt. A good product to try is Phosphate Edge™ by FSI Nutrition.

Muscle Building

The key secret to gaining weight is to shift the caloric balance. Calories consumed must be greater than calories expended on a daily and consistent basis to allow for permanent weight gain to occur. Scientists seem to be discussing muscle growth by two means: hypertrophy and hyperplasia. Hypertrophy is the actual growth of the muscle fiber in size and hyperplasia is the creation of new muscle cells. There is proof for both of these things occurring. Key supplements, good nutrition, and, of course, heavy lifting are the real keys to gaining muscle!

SPECIALTY SUPPLEMENTS

These cutting-edge sports supplements do not appear on the radar screen of most people, but they can have powerful, specialized effects on your body and help you build muscle and achieve your fitness goals much quicker.

Alpha GPC

What is it? Alpha GPC (L-alpha-glycerylphosphorylcholine) is an acetylcholine precursor derived from soy.

What does it do and how does it work? Alpha GPC has been shown in preliminary research to boost growth hormone (GH) levels and increase neurological function. Boosting GH levels can have major implications for muscle building and promoting optimal recovery from hard workouts, especially in individuals over the age of 40. Since Alpha GPC can boost levels of the neurotransmitter acetylcholine in the body, it can also help enhance mental focus and mental clarity, two good things to have during a workout. Alpha

GPC is a potent choline donor and the choline serves as a precursor for phosphatidylcholine, which can help protect cell membranes from damage.

What does the science say about it? In an Italian study, researchers concluded that individuals taking Alpha GPC had higher GH release. Yet another study published in 1992 called Alpha GPC a "cognitive enhancer," stating that its supplementation is an effective means to increase choline levels.

Dosage: This ingredient has good potential and is supplied by Chemi Nutraceutical as AlphaSize™. One plus is that even smaller amounts of Alpha GPC (150–400 mg) seem to boost GH levels, which makes it more cost effective.

Arginine AKG

What is it? Do the words "hemodilation" or "perpetual pump" mean anything to you? Well, they do to users of arginine alpha-ketoglutarate (arginine AKG; also known as arginine 2-oxoglutarate). It is claimed that this ingredient causes increased blood volume in muscle cells. Arginine AKG basically consists of the "conditionally essential" amino acid L-arginine bound to a "Krebs cycle intermediate," which may increase its absorption and target delivery to muscle cells.

What does it do and how does it work? Arginine has been researched extensively and has many beneficial effects, especially when it comes to cardiovascular health. Some research suggests it may help improve exercise performance, support protein synthesis, boost growth hormone levels at higher doses, and even help replenish glycogen (stored carbohydrate) stores post workout. Its main mechanism of action is boosting nitric oxide (NO) production, which helps promote its many effects. Nitric oxide is basically the muscle cells "signaling molecule." Boosting nitric oxide in muscle tissue can have many anabolic effects, including increased nutrient transport and vasodilation (increased blood flow). Arginine boosts NO by stimulating nitric oxide synthase, the enzyme that makes NO.

Theoretically, AKG is a glutamine precursor and may have a "glutamine sparing" effect in muscle tissue. This may be a side benefit of using this product, as glutamine (the most abundant amino acid in muscle tissue) can help athletes by boosting immune function, increasing cell volumization, supporting protein synthesis, and aiding in glycogen replenishment.

What does the science say about it? Some people claim that arginine AKG is the "the next creatine," but I think that is quite farfetched considering that over 200 studies confirming the use of creatine to boost exercise performance, strength, and muscle mass. Frankly, this product may have some benefits but it does not have anywhere near the clear research in humans (specifically athletes) that creatine does.

While solid and abundant testimonials from credible users should be considered, published clinical research is more important when determining if an ingredient really does work in promoting lean body mass, strength, and athletic performance. There was one small study showing arginine AKG supplementation increased bench press strength. Interestingly, though, the same study showed no significant differences in body mass, fat-free mass, or percent of body fat between exercisers taking arginine AKG and those taking a placebo. In another 2004 study, researchers found that nitric oxide supplementation didn't benefit healthy individuals.

The jury is still out on whether arginine AKG is as effective as some say it is. Questions that need to be answered include whether or not this ingredient is better than pure L-arginine (or other forms of arginine like arginine pyroglutamate or arginine hydrochloride) and whether or not increased blood volume and muscle pumps lead to greater strength and lean muscle mass over the long run.

Dosage: A good dose is generally 3–6 tabs (1 gram of arginine AKG per tab) about forty-five minutes before a workout or after meals.

Citrulline Malate

What is it? Citrulline malate is a compound consisting of citrulline, a non-essential amino acid, and malate, which is the ionized form of malic acid, a citric acid cycle intermediate that is important for energy.

What does it do and how does it work? Citrulline malate seems to enhance aerobic performance in exercising individuals and athletes. It also delays fatigue. The proposed mechanisms of actions include increased NO (nitric oxide) production (by increasing arginine levels in the plasma), increasing ATP and energy levels, and reducing lactic acid and ammonia buildup.

What does the science say about it? This nutrient has fairly good research behind it. A French study published in the *British Journal of Sports Medi-*

cine in 2002 showed that citrulline malate supplementation "resulted in a significant reduction in the sensation of fatigue, a 34 percent increase in the rate of oxidative ATP production during exercise, and a 20 percent increase in the rate of phosphocreatine recovery after exercise, indicating a larger contribution of oxidative ATP synthesis to energy production." This is all very good for hard-training athletes. Yet another French study showed that it had anti-fatigue properties by protecting against acidosis and ammonia buildup. Remember, lactic acid and ammonia buildup lead to muscle fatigue.

Dosage: Most of the research used 3–6 grams daily, preferably one dose an hour before training. A good source of citrulline malate can be found in H-Blocker by iSatori Technologies or NO-Xplode by BSN.

Mucuna Pruriens

What is it? The herb *Mucuna pruriens* is also known as velvet bean and contains the very powerful neurotransmitter precursor L-Dopa (the amino acid L-dihydroxyphenylalanine).

What does it do and how does it work? *Mucuna pruriens* has been shown to increase mental alertness and improve coordination, but the main reason athletes should consider this herb is increased growth hormone (GH) release. L-Dopa is a powerful GH releaser and *Mucuna pruriens,* which contains about 15 percent L-Dopa, can have powerful effects in this regard. Increasing GH levels can have profound effects on lean body mass and fat loss. This herb may also have blood sugar–regulating properties, but this is not established yet from clinical studies.

What does the science say about it? A 2004 study published in London showed that it had good effects in the management of Parkinson's disease via its L-Dopa content. The researchers even suggested that this natural preparation may be better than conventional L-Dopa treatments. Now this may not be directly related to athletes, but it does show the efficacy of the L-Dopa content in this herb.

Dosage: Taking *Mucuna pruriens* along with Alpha GPC before bedtime can help maximize GH release during sleep, allowing for better recovery and recuperation as well as stimulating more muscle growth. An effective dose of *Mucuna pruriens* is 600–700 mg (standardized to 15 percent L-Dopa), taken about thirty minutes prior to bedtime. Alpha Dopa by Pinnacle is a quality product containing a good amount of *Mucuna pruriens.*

Rhodiola Rosea

What is it? *Rhodiola rosea,* a Russian herb also known as golden root or arctic root, was one of the best kept secrets in the dietary supplement world. This herb is what's known as an adaptogen, a compound that allows your body to adapt to stress and normalize function. This herb has been shown to significantly allow for improvements in athletic performance.

What does it do and how does it work? The majority of research performed on *Rhodiola rosea* has been geared toward improving physical and mental performance. It has been shown to delay fatigue and improve energy utilization during exercise. Muscle proteins and glutamic acid levels are enhanced when taking this supplement. It has even been linked to increased creatine phosphate and ATP (energy) levels. All of this leads scientists to believe that this supplement may increase strength and lean body mass. Researchers speculate that *Rhodiola rosea* helps reduce the stress that occurs secondary to exercise by stimulating the parasympathetic nervous system, which causes relaxation (as opposed to the sympathetic nervous system, which causes stimulation).

What does the science say about it? The results of thirty-five years of intensive clinical studies on *Rhodiola rosea* performed at leading Russian and Scandinavian clinics show that this nutrient can help increase protein synthesis, remove ammonia from the blood and have a detoxifying effect, increase blood supply to the muscles and the brain, and improve athletic performance.

Dosage: A typical dose is 100 mg, taken three times daily, especially after a hard workout.

ZMA

What is it? ZMA® is a highly specific and unique vitamin/mineral combination. ZMA is a special combination of zinc, magnesium, and vitamin B_6. The zinc in this outstanding product is specifically formulated as zinc aspartate and zinc mono L-methionine, which makes it more bioavailable because of the two forms of chelates. The magnesium is also found in a chelated form bound to aspartate. In fact, the magnesium and zinc are bound together to the aspartate to enhance absorption. Absorption and usage of minerals is a key factor in receiving their many benefits

What does it do and how does it work? This powerful combination can have a positive impact on athletic performance and testosterone levels. Boosting the hormone testosterone can have many benefits including increased strength, lean muscle mass, and energy levels. Research conducted on athletes' strength shows that this precise combination of zinc, magnesium, and vitamin B_6 can increase total and free testosterone levels by 30 percent. Zinc is involved in the action of several hormones, including insulin, growth hormone, testosterone, and estrogen, and it is involved in more than 200 enzymatic reactions. Research has indicated that exercising individuals have a greater need for zinc. Magnesium is involved in over 300 enzymatic reactions in the body, including glycolysis, the Krebs cycle, creatine phosphate formation, nucleic acid synthesis, amino acid activation, cardiac and smooth muscle contractability, and, most importantly for strength athletes, protein synthesis. Vitamin B_6 (pyridoxine) is associated with a vast number of enzymes as a part of amino acid metabolism. It is necessary in glycogen catabolism to "unlock" carbohydrate energy and vitamin B_6 has also been shown to diminish the actions of certain catabolic steroids, such as glucocorticoid hormones (cortisol). This can boost the testosterone to cortisol ratio, which can lead to positive muscle-building effects.

What does the science say about it? A study published in *Medicine and Science in Sports and Exercise* showed that nightly supplementation with ZMA increased strength and power. A 1996 study showed that taking 30 mg of supplemental zinc daily by healthy men experiencing moderate zinc deficiency doubled their testosterone levels in six months.

Dosage: The best time to take ZMA is about thirty minutes prior to bedtime, usually at the recommended dose on the bottle.

Carnosine

New research is laying the path for an ergogenic aid that may eclipse the phenomenal success of creatine monohydrate. Carnosine (beta-alanyly-L-histidine), composed of two amino acids—histidine and beta-alanine—was discovered in 1900. Over the past 100 years, the focus of research has developed around assigning carnosine a biological role or function. The search has spanned the disciplines of human physiology, biochemistry, and even neurochemistry. But it wasn't until the 1990s that the first of two studies was released indicating its true nature with respect to exercise performance. What is carnosine's potential for performance enhancement?

To answer this and other questions, we interviewed the world's foremost authority on carnosine, muscle biochemist Mark J. Tallon, Ph.D., of the University College Chichester. Tallon received his master's degree in nutrition from the University of Liverpool, England, in 1990 and completed his Ph.D. in muscle biochemistry under the supervision of Professor Roger Harris, a leading creatine researcher and a carnosine specialist in his own right. Since the late 1990s, he has worked with Olympians in the area of nutritional biochemistry and applied sports nutrition. Tallon is the co-founder of CR-Technologies and the chief scientific officer of OxygeniX.com, which offers specialist nutritional advisory services to elite athletes and the general public interested in physique enhancement.

Stephen Adelé: *What led to your interest in muscle biochemistry?*

Mark Tallon: I have been a competitive athlete for some time and had the pleasure of working with some of the world's best athletes. I have also had an interest in muscle physiology from my early days in weight training. So, being in a situation where I can bring together both of these disciplines has been a fantastic opportunity. Over recent years, the field of muscle physiology and the application of nutritional aids to athletic performance enhancement have attracted some great funding and, as such, more research and indeed more researchers.

SA: *In which sports do you participate?*

MT: In my teens, I used to compete in many martial arts, including karate, and went on to work as a physiologist to the English National squad as well as for many ultra-endurance athletes. For the past few years, I have been actively involved in Ironman distance triathlons, which involves a 2.5 kilometer (km) swim, 180 km bike race, and a full marathon run. So, you can't really say I don't walk the talk when it comes to applied sports nutrition.

SA: *What led to your research of carnosine?*

MT: Following a master's degree in sports nutrition and many years of personal interest in the application of ergogenic aids to my own personal performance, I knew this was the area for me. Like everyone else, I was blown away by the change to the whole nutrition industry once creatine emerged, so I sought out the leader at that time in the field, Professor Roger Harris, formally of the Karolinska institute in Sweden and now Research Professor at University College Chichester, in England. In 1999, I was fortunate to secure a doctorate under his guidance in carnosine metabolism in human skeletal muscle. During this time, the issues of carnosine and muscle performance and other areas of a more pathological nature, such as age-induced muscle loss, were in their infancy.

SA: *What is the role carnosine has in muscle metabolism and, indeed, how could increased muscle stores increase performance?*

MT: As I mentioned, carnosine metabolism was only just beginning to be understood for its functional role in skeletal muscle function. Previously, its primary role had been thought to be as an antioxidant, although there were two studies—Parkhouse (1995) and Harris and Greenhaff (1998)—that started to lay the foundations of my doctoral work in human physiology. So, how might it affect performance? Well, carnosine is preferentially located in type II muscle fibers, which provide us with the fast-twitch characteristics needed to propel sprinters like Maurice Greene to world record excellence.

Carnosine is found in high amounts in the muscles of those exposed to prolonged and low muscle pH (higher acidity). This decrease in pH is not due to lactate per se, which you may have been told in the past, but rather to the production of hydrogen ions (H^+) as part of the process of energy release. As we work at higher intensities, we need an equal increase in our rate of energy production. For instance, in such events as an 800 meter sprint or intense weight training, this turnover is high and H^+ formation is multiplied accordingly. As hydrogen ions are released, intramuscular pH can begin to fall, leading to fatigue—unless we can prevent it.

How do we achieve this maintenance (buffering) of pH? Wouldn't it be fantastic if we had a system in place that can do this? Well, we do: the main intramuscular buffering system involves phosphates (one reason why creatine is effective), bicarbonate, and proteins, of which carnosine is a constituent. At the physiological pH at which muscle contraction occurs, carnosine can pick up H^+ and prevent, or should I say delay, the inevitable decrease in pH, increasing our ability to work harder for longer. The extent to which carnosine can delay acidosis is relative to its content in muscle, and this is where supplementation may eventually play a role.

SA: *What variation have you measured or observed in human subjects or athletes?*

MT: Well, many of my studies are in review at present, but what I can say is that we have biopsies from some extremely well-trained bodybuilders, and we have seen around a 50 percent increase in whole muscle carnosine, which could be much higher in type II muscle fibers due to the preferential distribution. This would have a huge impact on performance and resistance to high-intensity fatigue if we could achieve this through supplementation.

SA: *You suggested earlier that with increased muscle stores might come enhanced muscle function. How could this be achieved? Have you carried out dosing?*

MT: Supplemental carnosine is already sold in many health food stores but is promoted as either an antioxidant or an anti-aging agent. Yes, we have shown that carnosine can be elevated within skeletal muscle and have carried out a series of studies on different dosing regimes between 3 grams and 30 grams a day. The problem at the moment is the high cost of carnosine. We have also worked on the use of beta-alanine, guessing that it may be the limiting factor for carnosine synthesis. As with all supplements, it's not just the amount, but also the timing when you take them.

SA: *Are there any issues of safety on the use of carnosine?*

MT: Studies have found that there may be some parathesis (tingling sensations), which may be brought about by prostaglandin release. The negative health effects are unknown at this time, but carnosine is a well-known competitive inhibitor of taurine and has been used to deplete muscle taurine stores in cat muscle. The effect of this on muscle contractility is also unknown. What we do know is that relatively low doses of carnosine supplementation, similar to that found in the normal dietary experience of meat eaters, has revealed no negative effects in a variety of health markers. Evidence from liver or kidney function tests, cardiac function, and other related clinical data suggest that carnosine over the short-term (one month) is in no way detrimental to any of the above factors.

SA: *Have you taken any performance measures?*

MT: To date, we have looked at different measures of contractility using involuntary electrical stimulation of the muscle as well as some performance tests. With beta-alanine, there seems to be some positive effect. As for carnosine, we are still correlating our results. However, anecdotally I have taken it myself and for any high-intensity work it seems to work fantastically well. But endurance performance seems to show little effect—we will just have to wait for further clinical data. There was one study that showed a significantly higher mean power during repeated sprints in subjects with higher muscle carnosine concentrations.

SA: *What's happening biochemically to achieve "carnosine loading"?*

MT: Let's hit on a bit of carnosine science 101 briefly. When we eat a food containing carnosine, it gets hydrolyzed (broken down) to its constituent amino acids, namely histidine and beta-alanine, by the enzyme carnosinase, which is highly active in blood. These amino acids are then taken up into the muscle, where they are reassembled or resynthesized to carnosine by carnosine synthetase. We know little of the transport system at present and are still some years away from the knowledge we have on creatine transports.

SA: *While these concepts have not been fully verified in human research, you do have some preliminary evidence from animal studies. What do they tell us?*

MT: Although dietary studies are rare, restrictive diets involving removal of histidine from the diet for periods as short as twenty-four days and as long as twelve weeks show that muscle carnosine levels are reduced. As for beta-alanine, one well-designed study showed that feeding a combination of beta-alanine (100 mg per kg of body weight) and histidine (12.5 mg/kg) for thirty days increased muscle carnosine by 13 percent. More recent studies have shown a two- to fivefold increase in rat muscle carnosine with a diet consisting of 1.8 percent carnosine.

SA: *Do you think carnosine would be significantly depleted with exercise?*

MT: It depends on many factors, including duration and intensity. There have been a few studies that looked at intermittent exercise and showed a decrease in muscle carnosine levels. The main study, however, was seriously flawed, because they measured muscle as wet weight, and during exercise, you get a large change in muscle blood content, so the weight is elevated, yet carnosine contents are not. So, in comparison, it looks like you have a loss of carnosine. Another study repeated an even higher intensity exercise protocol and showed no significant change in dry muscle. In humans, however, we do not know—even if carnosine were lost into plasma, we could not measure it as the breakdown of carnosine to beta-alanine and histidine is so fast. Therefore, we would have to either look at muscle loss or the release of histidine and beta-alanine in plasma as predictors of loss. My guess is there will be little significant loss in human muscle, as well.

SA: *Can carnosine supplementation have value to a healthy person other than improving performance?*

MT: I have been so lucky over the past few years to work with Nicola Muffulli, a leading orthopedic surgeon, and Dr. Mark Tarnopolsky, who to many will not need an introduction due to his many contributions to the field of sports nutrition. In a recent study, we have shown a marked decrease in muscle carnosine stores in the elderly, which may in some cases lead to a loss of functional buffering capacity of 10 percent or greater. If we could reverse this through supplementation, we could possibly ameliorate the associated symptoms of strength loss in the elderly. Other recent areas of study on autistic children taking 400 mg of carnosine, twice a day, for twelve weeks showed significant improvement in behavior.

SA: *What might a vegetarian experience by taking a carnosine supplement?*

MT: I would certainly see a role for carnosine supplementation in the vegetarian population, where limited carnosine or its precursors (meats) are present in the diet. As with creatine and vegetarians, the lower the natural levels of carnosine, the bigger the response to supplementation and associated performance changes.

SA: *What are you researching now?*

MT: At present, we are furthering our understanding of the biochemical pathways for the synthesis of carnosine, as well as some novel delivery systems that may further enhance levels of uptake. We are also investigating the specifics of training-induced changes in muscle carnosine.

Beta-alanine supplementation seems to be the best way to increase carnosine levels in the body. Two recommended products that may boost carnosine from beta-alanine are Red Dragon™ by Muscle-Link, and H-Blocker by iSatori Technologies. H-Blocker (www.H-Blocker.com) is the most comprehensive formula available on the market with beta-alanine and l-histidine.

Creatine

Scientific facts about creatine are hard to come by: broadcast and print media, the Internet, product information, and other literature frequently contain statements concerning the supplement, with one report seemingly contradicting the next. Fortunately, in the midst of these mixed messages are voices of reason—university researchers such as Paul Greenhaff, Ph.D., Mark Tarnopolsky, M.D., Ph.D., Anthony Almada, M.Sc., and Richard Kreider, Ph.D., to name just a few—whose educated insight adds some clarity. Those of you who are either using creatine or are considering giving it a try will undoubtedly be interested in what the scientific literature and true experts have to say about its effects and its safety.

Creatine as a supplement has actually been around for a while. There are anecdotal reports that athletes were using creatine in Eastern Europe to aid exercise performance and there are similar reports about Bulgarian soldiers taking creatine, but there is no literature to support either contention. The first actual study demonstrating that creatine supplementation could increase whole-body stores was probably performed in the early 1930s.

How Creatine Works

During brief, explosive-type exercises, the energy supplied to "rephosphorylate" (combine the phosphates) of ADP (adenosine diphosphate) to form ATP (adenosine triphosphate, the basic form of energy used by cells) is determined largely by the amount of phosphocreatine stored in your muscles. As the phosphocreatine stores become depleted, performance is likely to rapidly deteriorate, due to the inability to resynthesize ATP at the rate required.

University studies have shown that by supplementing with creatine, you may increase your muscles' phosphocreatine pools by over 20 percent. And a 20 percent increase in phosphocreatine levels, according to research, theoretically might be expected to increase high-intensity exercise performance by at least 5 percent, due to an increased regeneration of adenosine triphosphate (ATP), which is exhaustively depleted during strenuous training but which is the only thing our bodies can use for energy. Increasing the availability of phosphocreatine serves to help ATP levels during intense exercise and accelerates the rate of ATP reynthesis following high-intensity, short-duration exercises.

Creatine Benefits Everybody

Creatine is not just for athletes seeking that "extra edge" in workouts—it may provide the edge needed for people from all walks of life to lead healthier, more energetic lives. Creatine supplementation, according to Dr. Mark Tarnopolsky of McMaster University, isn't just of benefit to weight trainers. A study published in the *Journal of Neurology* showed that creatine helped those suffering from neuromuscular conditions to improve their ability to perform high-intensity exercise by 10 percent to 15 percent. Current studies are now underway looking at the potential for creatine supplementation in the elderly, patients having joint replacements, and patients with muscular dystrophy. Dr. Tarnopolsky said each of these investigations looks promising.

In a recent review paper published in the *Sports Medicine,* the researchers stated that "activities that involve jumping, sprinting, or cycling generally show improved sport performance following creatine ingestion." New research on creatine shows some other benefits. In a 2003 study conducted at the University of Sydney in Australia, the researchers showed that creatine supplementation had a significant effect on working memory and intelligence—bigger and smarter, now that's a good combination. Creatine also has direct antioxidant effects, which means it can boost immune function.

Creatine Enhances Maximal Exercise Performance

Creatine researchers Dr. Greenhaff, Dr. Tarnopolsky, and Ronald Terjung, Ph.D., FACSM, recently addressed questions related to biochemical, physiological, exercise performance, and potential health effects and clinical applications of creatine supplementation. The panelists were unanimous in their agreement that short-term creatine supplementation of around 20 grams (g) per day for 5 to 7 days can lead to improved exercise performance: "Most of the studies indicate that creatine supplementation significantly enhances the ability to produce higher muscular force and/or power output during short bouts of maximal exercise in healthy, young adults."

According to Baylor University researcher Dr. Kreider, "Numerous studies have examined the effects of short-term creatine supplementation (5–7 days) on exercise performance. The majority of initial studies suggested that creatine supplementation can significantly increase strength, power, sprint performance, and/or work performed during multiple sets of maximal-effort muscle contractions. More recent studies have supported these observations."

In a 1992 study, Dr. Roger Harris demonstrates that combining creatine supplementation with exercise (i.e., taking creatine immediately following your workouts) may allow you to achieve enhanced creatine uptake and therefore an increased ergogenic effect. In this study, mean total muscle

Creatine's Performance-Enhancing Benefits

- Increased one-repetition maximum (IRM) and/or peak power.
- Improved vertical jump.
- Increased work performed during repetitive sets of maximal-effort muscle contractions.
- Enhanced single-effort sprint performance in sprints lasting 6–30 seconds.
- Enhanced repetitive-sprint performance (e.g., 6 (6-second sprints with 30-second rest).
- Improves high-intensity exercise performance in events lasting 90–600 seconds.
- Increases AT (anaerobic threshold) and maximal VO_2 (the ability of the body to transport oxygen to the muscles).

Source: Kreider, R.B., et al., "Creatine Supplementation: Analysis of Ergogenic Value, Medical Safety, and Concerns." *Journal of Exercise Physiology Online* 1:1 (1998).

creatine concentration increased by 37 percent when creatine was combined with exercise, as opposed to 26 percent with creatine supplementation alone.

Creatine Increases Muscle Size and Strength

A number of studies have evaluated the effects of creatine supplementation on muscle size and strength. According to a study recently published in the *Journal of Strength and Conditioning Research,* Dr. Kelly and colleagues reported that twenty-six days of creatine supplementation (20 g a day for four days, then 5 g a day thereafter) significantly increased body mass, fat-free mass, three-repetition maximum on the bench press, and the number of repetitions performed in the bench press over a series of sets in eighteen power lifters.

In another study published in *Medicine and Science in Sports and Exercise,* Dr. Kreider and colleagues reported that creatine supplementation (15.75 g a day for twenty-eight days) during off-season college football training promoted greater gains in fat-free mass in comparison to subjects taking a placebo. In a 1999 study published in *Medicine and Science in Sports and Exercise,* Dr. Volek and colleagues reported that twelve weeks of creatine supplementation (25 g a day for seven days; 5 g a day thereafter) during periodized resistance training increased fat-free mass, types I, IIa, and IIb muscle fiber diameter, one-repetition maximum squat and bench press, and lifting volume in nineteen resistance-trained athletes. Finally, in a recent edition of the *Journal of Strength and Conditioning Research,* Dr. Pearson and colleagues report that creatine supplementation (5 g a day for ten weeks) during resistance training promoted greater gains in measures of strength, power, and body mass with no change in percentage of body fat in 16 Division IA college football players during summer conditioning.

According to Dr. Kreider, "About 90 percent of long-term training studies report some ergogenic benefit with gains typically 10 to 100 percent greater than controls." In a comprehensive review of the scientific literature related to creatine supplementation, Dr. Kreider notes there are two main theories for the increased muscle size and strength from creatine supplementation. A third and more controversial theory related to creatine's effects on anabolic hormone levels has been proposed, but further research needs to be carried out to confirm these effects.

- **Enhanced Quality of Training**—Creatine in the muscle is an essential component to the production of ATP, the body's energy molecule. More available energy may allow for longer, more intense, and more frequent bouts of physical activity. Thus, creatine supplementation, studies show, may produce noticeable effects in muscle size and strength by enhancing energy reserves in the muscle cells.

• **Cell Volumization**—It is well-documented in the scientific literature that as creatine is taken up into the muscle cells, it also associates with water. "As more creatine is stored, more water may be brought into the muscle," says biochemist and creatine researcher Dr. Richard A. Passwater. "When muscle cell volume is increased, it is thought that this triggers more protein and glycogen synthesis, reduces protein breakdown (proteolysis) and increases muscle mass."

Although it has been hypothesized that the initial weight gain associated with creatine supplementation is primarily due to increased water retention, new research suggests otherwise. "A number of studies indicate that long-term creatine supplementation increases fat-free mass and/or muscle fiber diameter with no disproportional increase in total body water," states Dr. Kreider. "These findings suggest that the weight gain observed during training is most likely muscle mass."

• **Anabolic Hormone Increase?**—According to a team of researchers from Chukyo University in Toyota, Japan, creatine may in fact have direct anabolic properties due to its effect on enhancing human growth hormone secretion. Dr. J. M. Schedel and colleagues found that subjects who loaded with 20 g of creatine showed a "significant stimulation" of growth hormone between two and six hours after ingestion versus those who were given a placebo. The researchers concluded that, in resting conditions and at loading dosages, creatine supplementation mimics the response of intense exercise, which also stimulates growth hormone secretion. This, they say, could partly explain the dramatic muscle size and strength increases observed after creatine loading and should, along with other factors, be considered when investigating just how creatine works its magic.

Creatine Benefits Endurance Athletes

Although creatine supplementation does not appear to directly enhance aerobic-oriented activities per se, recent research has shown creatine supplementation may have a positive effect (upward of 30 percent increase) on the power production during short sprints within and at the end of an endurance exercise training session. "As I've been told by this type of athlete, at the end of the race they are actually running maximally," says Dr. Greenhaff. "And in that situation, creatine may indeed have a beneficial effect."

In one recent study in *Medicine and Science in Sports and Exercise*, researchers investigated the effects of a lower dosage (6 g per day) of creatine in twelve triathletes, ages 22–27, who had completed their season's competitions. Results of this study show supplemental creatine increased the triathletes' "interval power" performance by 18 percent, while their "endurance performance" was unaffected. That means the athletes were faster during the hill climbs and most "intense" portions of the endurance event. The results of this study and others offer evidence that cyclists and road-race runners, and endurance athletes in general, may benefit significantly from supplementing their daily nutrition program with creatine.

Creatine May Protect Against Sports-Related Concussions

Sports-induced head injury prematurely ended Hall of Fame quarterback Steve Young's career and likely precipitated the Parkinson's disease suffered by boxing legend Muhammad Ali. Lately, it seems to be occurring with unprecedented regularity, particularly in professional football. Statistics from the NFL commissioner's office suggest that football injuries to the brain occur at a rate of one every 3.5 games. Moreover, the U.S. Centers for Disease Control and Prevention in Atlanta says that more than 300,000 such injuries happen to people participating in sports or recreational activities every year. Stricter rules to increase safety have been implemented in recent years to help lessen the risk, but in sports such as football, boxing, and hockey—where hitting is a part of the game—anything short of not competing won't entirely prevent injury from occurring.

While eliminating the risk of concussion in contact sports seems out of the question, a new study suggests that creatine may actually help reduce the severity of head injuries. The study, published in a recent issue of the *Annals of Neurology*, shows brain damage may be reduced by 21 percent when creatine is taken three days before injury and up to 36 percent when taken five days before injury. Moreover, the researchers also discovered that supplementing with creatine four weeks before such an injury may reduce the severity by 50 percent.

"We believe this is a highly significant finding in the field of neurotrauma," says study author Dr. Stephen Scheff, a professor at the University of Kentucky College of Medicine. "We know of nothing to date that has shown this type of benefit in preventing serious neurotrauma." According to the researchers, creatine may work to protect against head injury by providing the brain cells' mitochondria—the "powerhouses" of the cells—with a reserve source of fuel to keep them energized after injury, thus preventing them from dying off.

"There are a number of athletes taking creatine, and they're taking it primarily to help build lean muscle and help them recover from short bursts of activity," says Dr. Scheff. "Now we find out they're also inadvertently protecting themselves, as well."

Dr. Scheff says researchers have often wondered why it is that NFL quarterbacks who've suffered so many concussions—such as former Dallas Cowboy Troy Aikman—have been able to play again shortly after sustaining an injury that would ordinarily keep someone sidelined for months. "We think the reason may be that 75 percent of professional football players take creatine," says Dr. Scheff.

Does Creatine Cause Muscle Cramping?

Many so-called experts have recommended avoiding creatine because it supposedly causes muscle cramps and strains. According to Dr. Kreider, who recently reviewed 76 such scientific studies directly related to creatine's ergogenic value and medical safety, proponents for this theory suggest that creatine supplementation may cause large fluid shifts into the muscle, serving to alter electrolyte status, promote dehydration, and increase thermal stress. "However," states Dr. Kreider, "No study has reported that creatine supplementation causes cramping, dehydration, or changes in electrolyte concentrations, even though some of these studies have evaluated highly trained athletes undergoing intense training in hot/humid environments."

For example, recently researchers examined the effects creatine had on the incidence of cramping and injury during preseason college football training in Division 1A athletes. According to the authors, creatine supplementation up to 15.75 g a day in hot and humid environmental conditions "does not increase the incidence of muscle cramping or injury and may, in fact, *reduce* the incidence of injury."

Another study performed in 2001 by Ball State University researcher Jeff Volek, Ph.D., came to a similar conclusion. In that study, Dr. Volek and colleagues examined the effects of creatine on men who exercised intensely in 97°F heat and 80 percent relative humidity—conditions supposedly ripe for creatine-caused muscle cramping. Even after receiving a loading dose of creatine (more than 20 g) and performing 30 minutes of intense cycling followed by three all-out 10-second sprints in such extreme conditions, "there were no reports of adverse symptoms, including muscle cramping," notes Dr. Volek.

The most common cause of reported muscle cramps, say the researchers, is not creatine supplementation but likely inadequate water and electrolyte ingestion. To avoid such problems, they recommend athletes consume at least 10 glasses of water per day.

Creatine in the Diet

Creatine is found in some foods, such as meats and fish, but according to Nottingham University researcher Dr. Paul Greenhaff, to increase athletic performance and boost lean body mass, creatine must be taken in concentrations that are not reasonably obtained from a whole-food diet. "Herring has a very high creatine store (about 3 grams of creatine per pound)," says Dr. Greenhaff. "That is probably the highest of the foodstuffs I know, but creatine is degraded during cooking." Thus, you would have to consume just less than 7 pounds of raw herring a day for five days to load your body with creatine. "I'd say you would struggle to get a large dose of creatine from foods," says Dr. Greenhaff.

Creatine in Whole Foods

Food	Creatine (grams/pound)	Food	Creatine (grams/pound)
Beef	2.0	Milk	0.05
Cod	1.4	Pork	2.3
Cranberries	0.009	Salmon	2.0
Herring	3.0	Tuna	1.8

Adapted from: Balsom, P.D., et al. "Creatine in Humans with Special Reference to Creatine Supplementation." *Sports Medicine* 18:4 (1994): 270.

Coffee and Creatine

Does coffee minimize creatine's effects? This theory has its roots in a 1996 study in which the authors compared the effects of oral creatine supplementation alone, and with creatine supplementation in combination with caffeine, on muscle phosphocreatine level and performance in nine healthy male volunteers. The study showed the usual ergogenic response to creatine supplementation. The authors remarked that their data show creatine supplementation to elevate muscle phosphocreatine and to markedly improve performance during intense intermittent exercise. This ergogenic effect, however, was completely eliminated by caffeine intake.

In the ensuing years, the interaction between caffeine and creatine was largely ignored and many people don't believe that caffeine has any adverse effects on creatine. However, the same laboratory has another study showing that caffeine intake overrides some of the effects of creatine

Vegetarians and Creatine Supplementation

It's been widely believed that creatine supplementation may be of greater benefit to those with low resting-muscle creatine and phosphocreatine stores, such as vegetarians (remember, creatine is found naturally in some meats, like beef and fish). To test this, scientists from the University of Saskatchewan and McMaster University randomly assigned a group of vegetarians and a group of nonvegetarians to receive a placebo or a creatine supplement and take part in heavy resistance training for eight weeks. Muscle biopsies taken before the study revealed that total creatine concentrations were nearly 10 percent lower in the vegetarian group.

According to the researchers, creatine supplementation in conjunction with weight-training exercise resulted in a 79 percent greater increase in phosphocreatine stores and a 169 percent greater increase in total creatine concentrations in the vegetarians compared to the nonvegetarians. Moreover, this translated into a significantly greater increase in type II muscle fiber area, suggesting a more dramatic response to muscle growth in vegetarians supplementing with creatine.

So, while these findings show that a vegetarian diet results in lower resting total creatine concentrations, creatine supplementation seems to promote greater increases in muscle phosphocreatine and total creatine stores in vegetarians, which may mean more dramatic increases in muscle size and strength.

on muscle mass and strength. Specifically, the researchers found that oral creatine supplementation shortens muscle relaxation time in humans by around 5 percent. This shortened muscle relaxation time, according to the researchers, may be important to the performance-enhancing action of creatine supplementation as well as power production during sprint exercise. Interestingly, the researchers also discovered that short-term caffeine intake, but not acute or intermittent caffeine intake, seems to *prolong* muscle relaxation time, thereby counteracting much of creatine's beneficial effects.

The bottom line is, if you're taking creatine, you might want to ease up on your daily coffee drinking and only consume caffeine intermittently before training.

Taking Creatine: Loading Protocols for Maximal Creatine Uptake

Creatine loading is a mechanism for increasing the creatine store of skeletal muscle, which in most people levels off in the at 140–160 millimoles per kilogram (mmol/kg) of dry muscle when using traditional loading protocols (i.e., 5 g of creatine taken four times a day for five days), according to research by Nottingham University professor Dr. Paul Greenhaff, who, with Dr. Eric Hultman, pioneered the study in this area in the early 1990s. By loading creatine, according to Dr. Greenhaff's and Dr. Hultman's research, you can increase muscle creatine uptake by about 25 percent. This is important because research shows the largest improvements in performance appear to be found in persons with the largest increases in muscle creatine concentration. In other words, the ergogenic (performance-enhancing) effect of creatine ingestion may critically depend on the extent of muscle creatine uptake during ingestion.

Since the early work of Drs. Hultman and Greenhaff, little has been done to advance the typical "5 grams four times a day" loading recommendations. But at least one leading creatine authority believes it's time to break with tradition—and he's got plenty of research to back him up. According to Professor Mark J. Tallon, Ph.D., of the University College of Chichester in the United Kingdom, new data is demonstrating that there is an alternative way to load creatine that may increase your muscle creatine by levels 30 percent greater than those achievable by traditional loading protocols.

According to Professor Tallon, if we *really* want to increase muscle crea-

CREATINE SUPPLEMENTS

Creatine Monohydrate

(available from many brands such as Phosphagen® by E.A.S.)

WHAT IS IT? This is creatine bound to a water molecule. It is the most widely used and researched form of creatine available today.

WHAT DOES IT DO? Enhances lean muscle mass, muscle size, strength, power, and short-term exercise performance.

DOSE: Load by taking 20–25 mg daily with grape juice for a week, and then maintain by taking 5 g daily, preferably after a workout.

Creatine Malate (di- and tri-)

(3-XL™ available from iSatori Technologies)

WHAT IS IT? This is two or three creatine molecules bound to malic acid, a Krebs' cycle intermediate that can further support energy production.

WHAT DOES IT DO? Human research is scarce, but theoretically it would have the same effects as creatine monohydrate and may mix/dissolve better in liquids.

DOSE: 5–10 g daily, preferably after a workout.

Creatine Magnesium Chelate

(available as Creatine Magnapower™ from Albion Labs)

WHAT IS IT? This is a patented amino acid chelate of creatine bound to the mineral magnesium, which is important for energy production and muscle function.

WHAT DOES IT DO? Increases strength, energy, and lean muscle mass. It may even increase cellular hydration and protein synthesis. It may also be better absorbed and retained by muscle tissue and cause less stomach discomfort.

DOSE: 5 g daily, preferably after a workout. No loading necessary.

Buffered Creatine

(available as Kre-Alkalyn™ from Sport-Specific Sciences)

WHAT IS IT? This is a patented buffered creatine monohydrate, which theoretically has a higher basic pH to make it stable in liquid.

WHAT DOES IT DO? Since this is basically "supercharged" creatine mono-hydrate, it would have the same effects. It is very stable, highly absorbable, and appears to cause no stomach discomfort.

DOSE: 2.5–5.0 g daily, preferably one dose before and one dose after a workout. No loading required due to its high absorption and stability rate.

Creatine Ethyl Ester

(available from BSN in their Cell-Mass product)

WHAT IS IT? This is creatine with an attached ester formed in a chemical reaction. This may make it more soluble and better absorbed.

WHAT DOES IT DO? In theory, it should have similar muscle-building effects of creatine monohydrate with better absorption, solubility, and greater uptake into muscle tissue over the short term. It may also cause greater stress to the liver, so be careful when using this product. There is little published research proving its effectiveness in humans.

DOSE: Low doses of 2–5 g daily may be beneficial. Take one dose after a workout or first thing in the morning on non-training days.

Effervescent Creatine

(available from FSI Nutrition)

WHAT IS IT? This is a self-dissolving buffered creatine citrate product.

WHAT DOES IT DO? There is not much published research, but it can have similar effects to creatine monohydrate. Its main benefit seems to be buffering the stomach acid to allow much less stomach discomfort and greater creatine absorption in the gut. In one pilot study, effervescent creatine was shown to be more effective in terms of anaerobic work capacity (exercise performance) than creatine monohydrate.

DOSE: One packet (providing 5 g of creatine) taken once daily after a workout or first thing in the morning on non-training days.

tine uptake dramatically, our focus needs to be on the cellular and molecular mechanisms regulating muscle creatine uptake, namely creatine receptor/transporter activity. You see, the transport of most nutrients in your body is mediated by a specific membrane-bound transport system. "Think of this system as walking over a bridge to get to work where you can carry out your job," says Professor Tallon. "Well, for creatine, the bridge it crosses before it can get to work is known as a creatine transporter." These creatine transporter proteins span muscle membranes allowing creatine to be transported directly into the muscle.

"When we investigate and dissect the research on nutrient uptake, it is the process of negative feedback/inhibition of these transport systems that control the levels of amino acids and related metabolites, including creatine, in muscle," says Professor Tallon. "This regulatory system seems to be directly and intrinsically linked to the concentration and time muscle cells are exposed to extracellular creatine."

So, what's the challenge with traditional loading regimens? Basic creatine pharmacology demonstrates that with a 5 g dose of creatine that passes intact through the intestinal lumen then into the bloodstream, you reach a peak concentration of creatine in the bloodstream of as much as or more than 840 umol/L after about sixty minutes. The problem is that the maximum capacity of creatine transport is reached at around 150 umol/L. Consequently, the traditional loading protocols may flood the creatine transport system, raising a red flag that may signal a rapid downregulation of creatine transport into the muscle.

According to Professor Tallon, there are two possible alterations to the creatine transport system that may result from traditional loading protocols. The first is the "acute response," which he says generally relates to the minutes and hours after creatine consumption and typically involves sodium changes across the cell membrane and decreased transport rates. The second is the "chronic response," which relates to alterations in the expression and number of creatine transporters on the plasma membrane.

"Looking at the typical loading phase developed back in 1992, the effects on human receptors over the first five days of loading have not been studied directly," says Professor Tallon. "What we do know, however, is that with high levels of intracellular creatine, a 50 percent decline in transporter activity has been observed." Consequently, over the five days of loading, we get less and less uptake of creatine into the muscle as transport speed decreases.

"This decrease in uptake in muscle eventually levels off at values of circa 140 mmol/kg (dry muscle)," he says. "This negative feedback is a bit of a pain because we probably make 80 to 90 percent of our total increase of muscle creatine in 48 hours, then it's really a case of maintaining this elevated level." What's more, not only do we start to get a decrease in the speed of uptake, "we get a double whammy because the body can recognize this new increase in creatine and starts to decrease the number of transporters on the muscle membranes."

A decrease in creatine transporters leads to less creatine for our muscles. How in the world do we get around this? "The key is in the first twenty-four to forty-eight hours of supplementation where creatine transporter activity is still very high, before the body has time to downregulate the speed of uptake or the expression of creatine transporter proteins," says Professor Tallon. "We need to keep plasma levels elevated to saturate the receptors consistently over this 48-hour window."

This approach will not elevate creatine to the same levels seen in typical loading protocols and as such will not saturate and cause a downregulation and expression of the creatine transporters. "To achieve this little trick we need to use small but regular creatine doses," he says. "Avoiding the 'peak and trough' approach demonstrated with regular creatine loading is the way forward. A program of 1.5 g to 2 g taken ten times a day will allow receptors constant access to creatine before the body can slow uptake down. In this way, we decrease the stress placed on the renal system and make available the best possible plasma creatine delivery system for enhanced uptake."

What does this elevation mean as far as performance and muscle-gain potential is concerned? "Well, the truth is nobody knows," says Professor Tallon. "But we could argue that there may be a further increase in both the ability to sustain high power outputs and to better tolerate muscle acidosis (the burning sensation we get toward the end of a set) through creatine's buffering effect. If the intensity and volume of our workouts can be prolonged, then it goes without saying increased muscle mass will be a definite byproduct of the appliance of science to our loading regimens."

To keep creatine receptor/transporter downregulation to a minimum, Professor Tallon recommends a regimen of 1.5 g to 2 g of creatine taken ten times a day for the first 48 hours, followed by a maintenance dose of 1.5 g to 2 g taken three times a day. The effects of adding insulin potentiators, such as the use of 4-hydroxyisoleucine, D-pinitol, or carbohydrates and protein, are relatively unknown, but may even further elevate uptake.

Do You Have to Load?

Can creatine content can be optimized without loading? "Yes, but it takes considerably longer," notes Dr. Greenhaff. "Lower-dose creatine supplementation (e.g., 3 g a day for two weeks) is less effective in the short-term at raising muscle creatine concentration than is a five-day regimen of

20 g a day. However, following four weeks of supplementation at this lower dose, muscle creatine accumulation is no different when the regimens are compared."

Loading for longer than five days seems to be unnecessary as studies show there's an upper limit to the amount of creatine and phosphocreatine our muscles can hold. In other words, you can't stockpile the stuff like a squirrel does nuts. Once muscle creatine accumulation has "maxed out"—which typically occurs during the initial four- to five-day loading period—creatine starts to spill out in the urine. Dr. Greenhaff's research shows that once creatine stores have been maximized, most humans simply do not need any more than 5 g of creatine per day to maintain optimal phosphocreatine reserves.

Certain Nutrients Enhance Creatine Uptake

In 1992, Dr. Roger Harris and colleagues from England's Nottingham University were among the first to show that creatine monohydrate supplementation (5 g, four to six times a day, for two or more days) significantly increased total muscle creatine content. It was further observed that while most people responded very well to creatine supplementation, about two or three out of 10 individuals don't—not because they were "immune" to its effects but because they just weren't achieving an optimal transport of creatine to muscle cells.

Several years later, other researchers demonstrated that virtually all subjects could become "responders" by ingesting 5 g of creatine monohydrate, followed thirty minutes later with 93 g of a simple carbohydrate (dextrose) drink (as found in Cell-Tech™ by MuscleTech), four times a day for five days, as this resulted in an increase in muscle phosphocreatine, creatine, and total creatine compared to creatine ingestion alone. These researchers also found that ingesting this creatine and simple carbohydrate combination dramatically elevated insulin concentrations, leading to the premise that creatine muscle uptake appears to be mediated in part by insulin.

Further investigation into this phenomenon has shown a number of ways a greater level of creatine uptake—and by consequence, a greater performance-enhancing effect from creatine—may be achieved short of consuming such large amounts of simple sugars and calories.

Creatine, Carbohydrates, and Protein

Recognizing the powerful "driving force" insulin has on creatine uptake, yet well aware of the downside of ingesting loads of sugar to stimulate its release, researchers from Nottingham University wanted to see if ingesting creatine in conjunction with 50 g each of both protein and simple carbohydrates would be as effective at potentiating insulin release and creatine retention as ingesting creatine in combination with almost 100 g of carbohydrates. Earlier research had shown that a protein and carbohydrate mix stimulates a release of insulin at levels far greater than just carbohydrates alone. So, the Nottingham researchers, led by Dr. G. R. Steenge, postulated that if protein were added to the mix, significantly fewer grams of simple sugars would need to be ingested to achieve optimal insulin levels.

The researchers recruited twelve men and had them consume 20 g (5 g, four times a day) of creatine per day in the following combinations: with 5 g of carbohydrates; with 50 g of protein and 47 g of carbohydrates; with 96 g of carbohydrates; or with 50 g of carbohydrates. The results showed that the release of insulin was no different when the protein/carbohydrate and the high-carbohydrate treatments were compared, but both were greater than the response recorded for the low-carbohydrate treatment. As a consequence, creatine uptake was increased by approximately 25 percent for both the protein/carbohydrate and high-carbohydrate treatments compared with the results of the placebo treatment. The researchers concluded that "the ingestion of creatine in conjunction with (about) 50 grams of protein and carbohydrates is as effective at potentiating insulin release and creatine retention as ingesting creatine in combination with almost 100 grams of carbohydrates."

Creatine and D-Pinitol

Since D-pinitol has been reported to have insulin-like properties, co-ingestion of D-pinitol with creatine may serve as a means of increasing creatine retention without having to ingest large quantities of simple carbohydrates and/or carbohydrates and protein. In a 2001 study appearing in *Journal of Exercise Physiology Online*, Dr. M. Greenwood and colleagues reported that creatine retention over a three-day loading period was significantly greater in subjects who consumed 5 g of creatine four times a day with a low dose of D-pinitol (500 mg, two times a day) compared with those who supplemented with creatine alone. Specifically, the percentage of supplemental creatine retained was about 83 percent in the creatine and D-pinitol group compared with just 61 percent in the creatine-only group. Interestingly, co-ingestion of creatine (5 g per day for four days) with a high dose of D-pinitol (500 mg, four times a day) did not appear to affect creatine retention, as subjects undergoing this protocol retained the same amount of creatine as the creatine-only group—61 percent.

Since D-pinitol is a relatively new discovery, the optimal dosage necessary to enhance the insulin-sensitizing effects in athletes is not clear. It would appear from this research that more is not necessarily better—stick with serving sizes of 500 mg twice a day when using D-pinitol with creatine (as found in Meta-CEL® from iSatori Technologies).

Creatine, 4-Hydroxyisoleucine, and Carbohydrates

Scientists have recently discovered that fenugreek seed (from the plant *Trigonella foenum graecum*) contains an unusual amino acid that may act as an insulin promoter. A team of French researchers, led by Dr. Christophe Broca, discovered that this amino acid, called 4-hydroxyisoleucine (4HI), stimulates insulin secretion in a glucose-dependent manner. This means that although 4HI by itself may not stimulate insulin secretion, you may be able to ingest fewer simple carbohydrates to achieve maximal insulin release and, by consequence, creatine delivery.

To date, three published studies support the efficacy of this compound for potentiating insulin response, thus conceivably increasing the efficiency of creatine transport. Although the specific research linking creatine transport and 4HI is in its preliminary stages, this compound seems to have good potential for optimizing the transport, and thereby performance-enhancing effects, of creatine.

Creatine's Long-Term Safety

Perhaps the most frequently expressed concern regarding creatine supplementation is the supposed lack of scientific knowledge regarding long-term side effects. While there's a definite need for more long-term, well-controlled clinical trials on creatine supplementation, it should be noted that there are over 70 years' worth of research on creatine, including trials lasting anywhere from five days to five years.

While many of those studies have been on creatine's ability to enhance performance in athletes and not its therapeutic effects, it should not be construed as unsafe. "Scientists in the field of exercise physiology follow the same rules of research as those scientists who investigate cures for disease," says South Dakota State University professor of exercise physiology Dr. Matt Vukovich, Ph.D. "If an exercise physiologist, or any other scientist for that matter, discovered creatine was harming individuals, it would be reported in the scientific literature."

In a recent study, Dr. Kreider examined the effects of long-term creatine supplementation on a 69-item panel of serum, whole blood, and urinary markers of clinical health status in athletes. Over a 21-month period, ninety-eight Division 1A college football players were administered creatine or non-creatine supplements following training sessions. Subjects who ingested creatine were given 15.75 g per day for five days, and an average of 5 g per day thereafter, in 5 g to 10 g doses. Fasting blood and 24-hour urine samples, as well as a host of other clinical data on markers of safety, were collected throughout the almost two-year study.

After extensive testing, Dr. Kreider stated, "Results indicate that long-term creatine supplementation (up to twenty-one months) does not appear to adversely affect markers of health status in athletes undergoing intense training in comparison to athletes who do not take creatine." In a separate review of over 500 research studies on the effects of creatine supplementation Dr. Kreider found that "no clinically significant side effects have been reported in these studies, even though many of them involved intense training in a variety of exercise conditions."

Muscle Cramping and Hydration

You've probably seen it before: an athlete is going strong and suddenly stops due to excrutiating pain in his or her muscles. They can no longer perform and need to sit out for a while because of pesky muscle cramps again. There are several things that can cause muscle cramping in athletes:

- Dehydration (especially while exercising in the heat)

- Mineral imbalances

- Lack of stretching

- Excessive loss of sodium and body fluids

- Vitamin deficiency

- Poor circulation

- Excess accumulation of lactic acid

Solutions

One of the best ways to stop or prevent a muscle cramp is to stretch thoroughly before, during, and after activity. Massaging the affected area can also help. Drinking a sports drink fortified with electrolytes, especially sodium and potassium, can help with recovery from muscle cramps. Making sure you are fully hydrated and consuming a good multivitamin/mineral formula daily is important. A good multimineral formula is Activate from MHP.

Water

Hydration is a very important aspect of any athletic program and water is an underrated but essential nutrient. Water has many functions in the body, including getting rid of toxins, transporting nutrients, cellular hydration or cell volumization (which can lead to a anabolic environment inside muscle cells), and supporting healthy skin function. According to research, dehydrating a muscle by as little as 3 percent can lead to a 12 percent decrease in strength. Plus, your muscle cells are about 70 percent water.

It is important to drink 1 to 1.5 gallons of pure water daily if you are exercising regularly. You should have clear urine as a sign that you are consuming a good amount of water daily. A more precise recommended daily dose for athletes is a minimum of 0.75 ounces per pound of body weight. So, a 200-pound athlete would need to consume 150 ounces of water daily—around 1.17 gallons, spread throughout the day (more during training, obviously).

Supplements

It is important to maintain a proper electrolyte balance (the proper balance of minerals in the body) to lower muscle cramping, dehydration, pH imbalance, and other unwanted effects of working out. Sports drinks can be very helpful in this regard. Look for a sports drink (like Gatorade or Powerade) that has potassium, sodium, and magnesium in it. Magnesium and potassium are especially important for helping to lower cramping. In fact, anyone that runs or cycles regularly should be taking 500–750 mg of magnesium (in the citrate or chelated form) daily to help reduce cramping and enhance energy levels. ZMA™, a special combination of zinc, magnesium, and vitamin B_6, may also help lower the incidence of cramping and possibly enhance recovery from endurance exercise. The amino acid taurine has also been shown in a few studies to reduce muscle cramping by protecting muscle cells from oxidative stress and exercise-induced damage. A good dose is 1–3 g, in two divided doses (before and after your workout).

Energy
and Endurance

Anyone who has worked for several hours straight with little sleep can tell you that they need more energy. Endurance athletes will tell you the same thing. It seems that everyone is looking to increase their energy levels. But how can one boost energy levels completely and sustain them throughout the day? To truly enhance energy levels, it requires increasing the three main parts of total body energy: mental energy, internal energy, and physical energy.

Mental Energy

Mental energy allows you to focus much better so you are sharp. How many times do you forget something you really needed to remember? Well, when mental energy is increased, forgetfulness is a thing of the past and you can also concentrate on key tasks and projects much better. There are many ways to increase mental energy. One is to boost levels of key neurotransmitters such as acetylcholine, dopamine, norepinephrine, and epinephrine, which allows signals from the brain to be sent more efficiently.

A powerful nutrient that can boost neurotransmitters is the amino acid L-tyrosine. This amino acid acts as a direct precursor to dopamine, norepinephrine, and epinephrine. This amino acid has been called the "focus" supplement, because it seems to enhance mental focus and mental clarity. This is especially useful before a workout or at the beginning of a long work day. A good dose is 500 mg to 1 gram taken 1–2 times daily, especially one hour before a workout. Energize by iSatori Technologies and L-Tyrosine by Kaizen are good products.

Another way to increase mental energy is to make sure there are no free radicals or other damaging compounds lurking in the brain. These destructive compounds can impair cognitive function, making you feel tired and lazy. Nutrients like vitamin C and gotu kolu seem to boost cognitive function by destroying these free radicals (an antioxidant effect). One study published in the *American Journal of Epidemiology* in 1998 showed that vitamin C protects against cognitive impairment. A study on gotu kola conducted in India concluded that it has cognition-enhancing effects through an antioxidant mechanism of action. A good dose is 1,000 mg of vitamin C and 180 mg of gotu kola in divided doses daily.

Caffeine also seems to boost brain function and focus in exercising individuals and it also reduces early morning sleepiness when taken at a fairly low dose. There is a compound in the brain called adenosine that slows down neuron activity. Caffeine blocks adenosine receptors, brain activity becomes heightened, and a stimulation effect occurs (as many coffee drinkers have experienced far too often).

Internal Energy

Internal energy requires thermogenesis (an increase in heat production), which leads not only to fat-burning effects but also to increased energy levels. The compound Bioperine® has been shown to increase thermogenesis and thereby increase energy. Take 5 mg twice daily. We know that green tea extract has powerful immune system supporting benefits, but newer research suggests that it also increases metabolism and can boost energy. Take 600–700 mg daily. Caffeine is another compound that can support a healthy metabolism and increase internal energy levels.

Physical Energy

Physical energy is also a must when looking to boost overall energy levels. This has to do with adapting to stress more efficiently and increasing ATP (cellular energy) levels in the body. Herbs such as ginseng and *Rhodiola rosea* have been shown to increase aerobic endurance and ATP levels in the body. They work as adaptogens, allowing the body to better adapt to stress as needed. Research on *Rhodiola rosea* has shown its usefulness in improving physical and mental performance. Take 100 mg three times daily. Caffeine again plays a role in physical energy by helping release more calcium from the sarcoplasmic reticulum, leading to greater muscle contraction and energy.

Energy Drinks

Energy drinks are a staple on the fitness programs of many people. These drinks are carbohydrate containing beverages that have some specialty ingredients specifically designed to increase energy levels. Most of these drinks are carbonated and taste like a citrus-type soda. Energy drinks start with simple carbohydrates: some contain glucose and/or sucrose, while others mainly have high-fructose corn syrup as their carbohydrate/sugar source. These drinks are filled with sugar, so they are definitely not for those on a strict fat-loss diet or for anyone following a low-carbohydrate lifestyle.

Carbohydrates can convert into glucose (blood sugar) and increase energy levels as glucose produces energy in the body. In fact, some research indicates that carbohydrates, and specifically glucose, can improve mental function—falling glucose levels lead to diminished cognitive function. Glucose is especially important during times of stress or high cognitive load. That is why these drinks contain a high amount of sugar to increase blood glucose levels. Carbohydrates are also necessary for endurance athletes to increase energy levels during times of training and competition.

Sucrose is commonly referred to as table sugar and is a disaccharide consisting of both glucose and fructose. Fructose is a more slowly absorbed carbohydrate found in fruits (fruit sugar). High-fructose corn syrup is a highly refined sugar consisting mainly of dextrose (glucose) and other disaccharides. It has been enzymatically treated and is a low-cost carbohydrate that has good stability in liquid. It is probably the lowest grade of the "energy yielding" carbohydrates but since it is cheap, many manufacturers use it.

Another major energy-boosting component of energy drinks is caffeine, which is sometimes found in its herbal version, guarana or kola nut. Most of these energy drinks have about as much or a little less caffeine than a regular cup of coffee. You may want to contact the manufacturers and ask them for a laboratory analysis of caffeine content in their drink to make sure you are getting what they claim.

The amino acid taurine is also found in energy drinks. Taurine is the second most abundant amino acid in muscle tissue (next to L-glutamine). It has some antioxidant and insulin-mimicking properties. It can help protect cells (including brain cells) from toxic damage. Taurine may also help prevent or decrease the cramping sometimes associated with beta-adrenergic agonists like synephrine.

Key B vitamins found in these drinks can act as enzyme cofactors involved in energy-producing reactions. For example, vitamin B_6 can help break down stored energy (glycogen) into usable energy. Herbs like ginseng and *Ginkgo biloba* are also found in some energy drinks to promote optimal mental function and allow the body to better adapt to stress.

Any healthy adult looking to boost energy levels or increase focus during certain times of the day may benefit from consuming energy drinks. Endurance athletes looking for an energy boost before a big race or training may also consider using them.

Dosage: Up to two cans daily can be consumed as needed for energy. A good time to take these drinks is in the morning so you can start the day focused. It may be a good idea to take a few weeks off of these drinks after twelve weeks of continued use. Do not use these drinks close to bedtime as they may interfere with sleep. Taking them on an empty stomach can enhance their effects and is preferred. Good ones include Red Bull, Monster, and Rock Star. Try their sugar-free versions so you can avoid unnecessary calories.

Sports Drinks

Sports drinks are specifically for sweating athletes who are exercising vigorously (and losing minerals and nutrients), not for the average individual looking for an energy boost. Maintaining sustained energy levels is essential to sports success. The science of sports drinks has certainly advanced since the days of sugar water! These products now contain many proven ingredients that can boost exercise performance and enhance recovery. But which products work best? When should these products be taken? Is there clinical research to support their use? And what about hydration and electrolyte balance?

First, let's look at some basic facts about carbohydrate and energy metabolism. Carbohydrates, specifically glucose, are an important energy source for many human tissues, including skeletal muscle. It would not be practical or efficient for your body to store significant amounts of glucose in solution, so carbohydrate reserves are stored in the form of the branched-chain polysaccharide called glycogen. Two-thirds of glycogen is stored in muscle tissue and one-third is stored in the liver. The muscle glycogen is what is important in providing energy to endurance athletes and fitness enthusiasts. Glycogen can be converted into glucose to provide energy to working muscles. This process can be circumvented and glycogen can be spared if a carbohydrate-containing solution is ingested during exercise. Another important point to remember is that for every gram of glycogen stored in the muscle tissue, there are three grams of water stored with it. This is important for hydration.

There have been many studies conducted showing the positive benefits of feeding during exercise. This is mainly in liquid form as liquids are better absorbed than solid foods, especially when exercise is being performed. Solid foods are not recommended during aerobic exercise as they may cause dehydration due to the digestive process. Plus, since they are not absorbed into the bloodstream as fast, they can't provide a quick burst of glucose like sports drinks. By the way, feeding during aerobic exercise can be beneficial when exercise is longer than thirty minutes. Exercise less than thirty minutes may not be impacted as much by the use of sports drinks or other workout aids during exercise. Consuming 12–16 ounces of water is one of the best things to do during exercise lasting under thirty minutes. Some research suggests that a 3 percent decrease in body water causes a 12 percent loss of strength.

The moral of the story is to drink plenty of water before, during, and after exercise. According to research conducted at the Australian Institute of Sport, adding flavor to a sports drink is known to enhance fluid intake during exercise. The researchers also found that flavored sports drinks cause better fluid balance than water alone and that the energy (carbohydrate) content of the drink is relatively unimportant in determining fluid intake.

Choosing a Sports Drink

So which sports drinks are best? According to a 2000 study published in *Sports Medicine*, researchers concluded that "there is little evidence that any one sports drink is superior to any of the other beverages on the market." Some important things to look for in a sports drink, according to another study published in the same journal in March 1998, are osmolality, carbohydrate concentration (5 to 7 percent), and carbohydrate type (multiple transportable carbohydrates are preferable). Osmolality, the concentration of particles in solution, increases with dehydration and decreases with overhydration.

There are many types of carbohydrates found in sports drinks, including maltodextrin, glucose, dextrose (which is basically glucose), sucrose (which is glucose plus fructose), fructose, glucose polymers, and high-fructose corn syrup (which is dextrose). The type of carbohydrate is important to its performance-enhancing benefits. It is important to get high-glycemic carbohydrates (like dextrose or glucose), which raise blood sugar levels quickly and provide a burst of energy. It is also important to get low-glycemic carbohydrates (like fructose), which are absorbed slower to provide sustained energy. However, too much fructose in sports drinks can cause an upset stomach.

Look for a combination of these carbohydrates in a sports drink. Maltodextrin is called a glucose polymer and a complex carbohydrate, but it has a high glycemic index and impacts blood sugar levels very quickly. This type of carbohydrate is great to take after a long run or bike ride to help replenish energy stores. In fact, sports drinks in general should not only be taken during exercise but also within twenty minutes after exercise to enhance the recovery process. A carbohydrate called galactose (glucose + lactose) is also showing up in sports drinks. This type of carbohydrate is easily absorbed and doesn't cause a massive blood sugar spike.

Another important thing that sports drinks provide are electrolytes. It is important to maintain an electrolyte balance (the proper levels of minerals in the body) to lower muscle cramping, dehydration, pH imbalance, and other unwanted effects. Look for a sports drink that has potassium, sodium, and magnesium in it. Magnesium and potassium are especially important, especially in helping to lower cramping. In fact, anyone that runs or cycles regularly should be taking 500–750 mg of magnesium (in the citrate or chelated form) daily to help reduce cramping and enhance energy levels. ZMA™ (a special combination of zinc, magnesium, and vitamin B$_6$) may also help lower the incidence of cramping and possibly enhance recovery from endurance exercise.

There are several "designer" ingredients that are found in engineered sports drinks that may enhance exercise performance. Vitargo® (Carbamyl) is a powerful high-molecular-weight carbohydrate from potato starch that may dramatically increase glycogen storage, according to clinical research on this product. It is a complex sugar-free carbohydrate available from Nutrex Research. The BCAAs (branched-chain amino acids) leucine, isoleucine, and valine may help delay muscle fatigue and prolong exercise, especially in the heat, when taken during a workout.

Antioxidants such as vitamin C, vitamin E, selenium, green tea extract, and others can help stop damaging free radicals, which is helpful during training when free radicals are being produced at a high rate. One study published in the *International Journal of Sports Medicine* in 2001 and conducted with ultra-marathoners clearly showed that vitamin C supplementation helped lower levels of the catabolic hormone cortisol secondary to the intense aerobic exercise. The study also showed enhanced recovery and recuperation. Try to get all of these antioxidants in liquid form for optimal absorption during a workout. There is a dietary supplement called ribose (a pentose sugar) that had some great potential as an energy booster, but the average results and expense of the product were disappointing. Carbogen™ (Triarco) is an enzyme blend that can help digest the carbohydrates in a sports drink so they are better utilized.

Many sports drinks contain nutrients such as L-carnitine and caffeine to maximize fat utilization (thus providing a good long-term energy source) and promote exercise endurance. Another important factor in supporting endurance is getting enough oxygen to working muscles. Low-carb sports drinks often contain supplements that increase blood flow and oxygenation to muscles, such as *Rhodiola rosea* and *Cordyceps*. These herbs can be very helpful in supporting long-term endurance activities.

Some sports drinks contain an endurance-boosting nutrient called glycerol, a colorless, odorless, sweet-tasting nutrient. It is technically a trihydroxy alcohol found naturally as the backbone of triglycerides in the body. It does not cause any significant blood-sugar response and seems to be eliminated from the body mostly unused. Glycerol has been shown to enhance athletic performance and cause "hyperhydration" when consumed with water (above and beyond water alone). This hyperhydration helps keep the body cooler during exercise. Glycerol does contain 4.3 calories per gram, so keep that in mind.

Many sports drinks also contain B vitamins, such as vitamin B_6, which can help boost energy levels. The coenzyme form of vitamin B_6 is associated with a vast number of enzymes, the majority of which are a part of amino acid metabolism. Vitamin B_6 is necessary in glycogen catabolism to "unlock" carbohydrate energy and it has also been shown to diminish the actions of certain catabolic steroids, such as cortisol.

Some top-notch sports drinks on the market include Accelerade® from Pacific Health Labs and G-Push®. Follow the dosing instructions on the label.

Insulin Management: Blood Sugar Regulating Supplements

I s insulin good or bad? Many people talk about controlling blood sugar levels and hence insulin levels to lower fat storage, reduce cravings, and sustain energy levels. Some diets have you cut out carbohydrates altogether to minimize and control insulin levels. Can insulin help you build more muscle mass or will it cause more fat storage? Insulin is a hormone that has been discussed heavily in the bodybuilding and health communities. It's time to set the record straight and find out more about this intriguing hormone and the supplements that can help you positively manipulate it.

What Is Insulin?

Let's dive into the functionality of insulin, including biochemistry, and see exactly how it works in the body and its metabolic consequences. Insulin is a peptide hormone that is released from the beta cells of the pancreas. It is released due to a rise in blood sugar levels that is induced mainly by eating carbohydrates and to a lesser degree by some amino acids in protein sources. This hormone is primarily responsible for the direction of energy metabolism after eating. Insulin helps regulate blood sugar levels and keep them in the range of 75–120 mg/dl (milligrams per deciliter). Individuals with metabolic disorders such as type I and type II diabetes mellitus cannot endogenously produce insulin so insulin shots are necessary (type I) or their bodies cannot use insulin properly and they may have insulin insensitivity (type II).

Insulin binds to specific receptors in cell membranes and helps drive glucose into the cell. Normally, the cell membranes are impermeable to glucose, but when a cell receptor is activated by insulin, the membrane allows for a rapid entry of glucose into the cells. Insulin helps activate glycogen synthase, an enzyme that helps make glycogen, a form of sugar, to be stored in muscle tissue (two-thirds of glycogen is stored in muscle tissue while one-third is stored in the liver). Liver glycogen is mainly used to help keep blood sugar levels stable. Insulin also allows cell membranes to become more permeable to certain amino acids, creatine, and some minerals.

Insulin causes glucose transport (GLUT) proteins to increase their activity, allowing for increased glucose uptake by muscle cells. Two of these transporters have been found in skeletal muscle: GLUT 1, which is present in low levels, and GLUT 4, which is the major isoform in muscle and is responsible for the increase in glucose transport in response to insulin and muscle contractions. It is believed that both insulin and exercise stimulate the translocation of GLUT 4 transporters from an intracellular pool to the plasma membrane of skeletal muscle. That is, exercise (muscle contraction to be specific) and insulin stimulate an increase in glucose uptake by muscle. There is ample evidence which suggests that exercise during a recovery period impedes glycogen synthesis, so you should refrain from any cardiovascular work right after resistance training. It may inhibit glycogen resynthesis and not let you recover from your weight-training session properly.

Although insulin helps dispose of blood glucose by storing it as glycogen in muscle tissue and the liver, it can also convert the excess to fat. Insulin is truly a double-edged sword due to this effect. Insulin seems to increase fat storage and fatty acid synthesis by activating the activity of lipoprotein lipase enzyme and acetyl CoA decarboxylase. What many people don't know is that insulin supports amino acid uptake into muscle tissue as well, allowing the muscle cells to have more amino acids available to help in the growth and recovery process. So, you have a hormone that can enhance glycogen levels in the muscle cells, thereby creating a more favorable environment for growth by causing cell volumization or cellular swelling (for every gram of glycogen stored in the muscle cell, there are 3 grams of water stored as well). This can have a hydrating effect on the muscles and also create more stored energy to be used later. Plus, some athletes report a better "pump" when using insulin-boosting supplements.

Insulin's opposing hormone is glucagon, which is activated when blood sugar levels are too low. This hormone can break down muscle tissue and reduce glycogen stores so it is important to control it.

Insulin release has also been shown to help transport more creatine into muscle tissue. It is theorized that taking "insulin-mimicking" supplements can help creatine transport as well. More research definitely needs to be done on these compounds to clarify their effects on creatine transport.

Using Insulin to Your Advantage

So, how do you use insulin to your advantage and minimize its fat-storing effects? First of all, it is important to raise and lower insulin levels at different times during the day. For example, insulin sensitivity is high first thing in the morning and right after a workout. Knowing this, it is important to maximize the use of insulin to drive nutrients into muscle cells during these key times (it is a good idea to take creatine at these two times to maximize absorption). Spiking insulin levels after a workout by consuming simple carbohydrates and protein (preferably in a liquid form) can block the catabolic effects of the hormone cortisol and allow for key nutrients to replenish muscle cells. Nutrient uptake is very high after a workout due to heightened enzymatic activity and, as mentioned previously, higher insulin sensitivity. Causing a spike in insulin levels after a workout can also enhance protein synthesis and lower the breakdown of protein secondary to weight training.

Bottom line—Take a good high-carbohydrate/moderate-protein drink 15–20 minutes after a workout session. Just like there are times you want to spike insulin levels to maximize nutrient uptake, there are also times you want to lower insulin as much as possible to prevent fat storage from occurring. One of these key times is at night before bedtime. Spiking insulin levels near bedtime can actually decrease or even suppress growth hormone (GH) levels (high insulin levels block GH, which is why GH levels are higher after a fasting state of 2–4 hours because insulin levels are lower). This can in turn lower the recovery process as well as impede muscle growth. Since metabolism is generally slower at night, eating carbohydrates or certain amino acids (like the branched-chain amino acids leucine, isoleucine, and valine) that can cause an insulin response may allow for greater fat storage at this time. It is a good idea to lower carb intake at night and eat more fiber and protein.

Supplements for Optimal Insulin and Blood Sugar Levels

These supplements help stabilize blood sugar levels and support insulin release, so it is a good idea to take them with carbohydrate-containing meals. Dosages need to be adjusted for body weight.

Alpha-Lipoic Acid

What is it? Alpha-lipoic acid (thioctic acid) is a sulfur-containing antioxidant produced naturally by the body and can be found in foods such as liver, brewer's yeast, and potatoes. It is found in the mitochondria of cells.

What does it do and how does it work? Alpha-lipoic acid is a unique and powerful fat- and water-soluble antioxidant, an insulin mimicker, and it plays a key role in producing cellular energy. It is actually prescribed in parts of Europe for blood sugar disorders! In the metabolic cycle, alpha-lipoic acid acts as a coenzyme in the production of energy by converting carbohydrates into energy (adenosine triphosphate or ATP). In a series of steps, carbohydrates are broken down into sugars, which results in pyruvic acid; this in turn breaks down to an enzyme complex that contains alpha-lipoic acid. The end result is more energy. This action is considerably important for people who exercise, since higher levels of energy may be desired and often required. Alpha-lipoic acid is a necessary component of the energy transport reactions that allow for glucose to be metabolized into energy (ATP). Alpha-lipoic acid can also help your fitness efforts by normalizing blood sugar levels, while metabolizing sugar into energy and increasing energy levels. Because it can help regulate blood sugar levels, it is sometimes called an insulin-mimetic compound.

What does the science say about it? Alpha-lipoic acid has been well studied in diabetics, especially for its positive role in diabetic neuropathy. Research shows that it enhances insulin sensitivity, glucose transport, and acts as an insulin-mimicking agent. It acts as a universal antioxidant and has synergistic effects with vitamins C and E. According to a 2006 study conducted at the University of Arizona College of Medicine, alpha-lipoic acid along with exercise has been shown to enhance insulin action in insulin-resistant skeletal muscle. An Italian study published in 1995 showed it may enhance muscle performance by increasing energy levels. Other studies show it may reduce exercise-induced oxidative stress.

Dosage: A typical dose of alpha-lipoic acid is 100 mg, taken three times daily with meals (although some research shows benefit with up to 600 mg daily). A single dose taken an hour before training may be beneficial. The R-lipoic acid form (which is the naturally occurring version) seems to have greater bioavailability.

Chromium

What is it? Chromium (Cr) is a trace mineral that comes in various forms, including chromium picolinate and the chromium polynicotinate form, which seems to be better absorbed.

What does it do and how does it work? Chromium is needed for normal protein, fat, and carbohydrate metabolism. It is also important for energy production and plays a key role in regulating appetite, reducing sugar cravings, and increasing lean body mass. Chromium helps insulin metabolize fat, turn protein into muscle, and convert sugar into energy. The primary function of chromium is to potentiate the effects of insulin and thereby enhance glucose, amino acid, and fat metabolism. It enhances insulin sensitivity. Exercise induces chromium losses in athletes and may lead to chromium deficiency, resulting in impaired insulin function. The biologically active component of glucose tolerance factor (GTF), which potentiates insulin activity and is responsible for normal insulin function, is dependent on chromium. Due to excessive chromium loss during vigorous exercise, athletes may have an increased requirement for chromium, since insulin's effects on carbohydrate, fat, and protein metabolism are dependent upon the maintenance of adequate chromium stores.

What does the science say about it? Chromium polynicotinate (or nicotinate) has been shown to ameliorate type II diabetes, reduce hypertension, help decrease fat mass and increase lean body mass, as well as reduce weight. A 1997 study conducted at the University of Texas showed that chromium polynicotinate supplementation caused significant weight loss in conjunction with exercise and it also helped modify insulin response to a glucose load. Another study at the Georgetown University Medical Center showed similar fat loss effects in overweight women. Other animal research has shown that chromium may have positive effects for syndrome X (metabolic syndrome or insulin resistance syndrome). Research published in the *Journal of Psychiatric Practice* (September 2005) showed that 600 mcg of elemental chromium (chromium picolinate) helped suppress appetite and reduced carbohydrate cravings.

Dosage: Taking 200 mcg of chromium, 2–5 times daily, can be useful. Taking 400 mcg of chromium after a weight-training session can further enhance insulin sensitivity and improve nutrient transport. A case can be made for using either chromium picolinate or chromium polynicotinate, as there is research to support both of these forms of chromium. Since dietary chromium is poorly absorbed, it would be beneficial to use one of these supplemental forms.

Gymnema Sylvestre

What is it? *Gymnema sylvestre* is a woody, vine-like plant that has been used for centuries in Ayurvedic medicine. The medicinally active parts of the plant are the leaves and the roots.

What does it do and how does it work? *Gymnema sylvestre* has an active compound called gymnemic acid made up of molecules that are similar to that of glucose molecules. Those molecules fill the receptor locations on the taste buds for a period of one to two hours, thereby preventing the taste buds from being activated by any sugar molecules present in food. Similarly, the glucose-like molecules in gymnemic acid fill the receptor locations in the absorptive layers of the intestine, which significantly reduces the metabolic effects of sugar by preventing the intestines from absorbing those sugar molecules during the digestive process. Due to the change in the absorption of sugar, there is a consequent change in the blood sugar level.

What does the science say about it? Clinical tests show that regular use of *Gymnema sylvestre* over a period of three to four months helped to reduce glycosuria, the appearance of carbohydrates in urine. Recent clinical trials conducted in India have shown that an extract of *Gymnema sylvestre* is useful for controlling blood sugar.

Dosage: The recommended dose of *Gymnema sylvestre* is 150 mg (standardized to 75 percent gymnemic acids), taken 3–4 times daily with carbohydrate-containing meals (especially sugar).

Corosolic Acid

What is it? Corosolic acid is a unique triterpene compound extracted from the leaves of the plant *Lagerstroemia speciosa*. The leaves of *Lagerstroemia speciosa* are used in Southeast Asia as an herbal remedy for several ailments, including diabetes.

What does it do and how does it work? Corosolic acid acts as a glucose transport stimulator. Several types of glucose transporters are known to exist in cell membranes of mammalian tissues. They are important in regulating the levels of intracellular glucose. Glucose transport is one of the most important functions of all cells in order to acquire energy. Modifications of the activity of glucose transport would cause several physiological effects, such as lowering blood glucose levels. Until now, only a few compounds have been known to affect glucose transport activity. Corosolic acid is called a phyto-insulin or insulin-like substance because of its ability to aid in blood sugar regulation. Insulin increases this glucose transporter activity. Because of its ability to mimic the actions of insulin, corosolic acid may aid in creatine (an amino acid important for muscle building) transport into muscle tissue. It can also increase energy levels by increasing carbohydrate stores (glycogen) in the muscle.

What does the science say about it? Dr. Kazuo Yamasaki, Professor of Pharmaceutical Science at the Hiroshima University School of Medicine, in Japan, studied the beneficial effects of corosolic acid, found in the supplement Glucosol™ (Opti-Pure). His studies indicated that corosolic acid is an activator of glucose transport, which results in hypoglycemic effect or low blood sugar level. Other research published in the *Journal of Ethnopharmacology* in 2003 showed that it has anti-diabetic effects in type II diabetics.

Dosage: For weight loss, a typical dose is 16 mg of corosolic acid, taken 2–3 times daily, with one of the doses taken after a workout.

D-Pinitol

What is it? D-pinitol is a methyl ester of D-chiro-inositol, an active principle of the traditional antidiabetic plant *Bougainvillea spectabilis*. It is contained in pine wood and legumes, but is derived from soy for manufacturing supplements.

What does it do and how does it work? D-pinitol has been shown to decrease blood sugar levels and free fatty acid levels—useful for someone trying to lose body fat. It has been patented by Humanetics for several uses, with one as a supplement for the therapeutic treatment of insulin-resistant type II diabetes. Two of D-pinitol's most significant effects for athletes are its ability to increase glucose uptake by the muscle cells and its ability to enhance glycogen storage (carbohydrate storage in the muscles). This can lead to greater energy and more stable blood sugar levels. It has been shown in clinical research that Pinitol can improve insulin function by increasing insulin sensitivity, thereby allowing insulin to work more efficiently.

What does the science say about it? A 2001 study published in the *Journal of Exercise Physiology* showed that D-pinitol supplementation helped enhance creatine retention. There was a synergistic effect when D-pinitol was taken with creatine. This is good news for anyone who wants to avoid taking high doses of sugar with creatine to enhance creatine transport and retention. In fact, the researchers of this study, including noted scientists like Richard Kreider, Ph.D., mentioned that "results suggest that ingesting creatine with low doses of D-pinitol may augment whole body creatine retention in a similar manner as has been reported with co-ingestion of high levels of carbohydrate or carbohydrate and protein." A 2000 study published in the *British Journal of Pharmacology* concluded that D-pinitol exerts insulin-like effects that would improve glycemic control and hence optimize blood sugar levels.

Dosage: A good dose of D-pinitol is 250 mg, taken 2–3 times daily with meals, and one dose with post-workout creatine. Nitro-Tech® by Muscle-Tech and Meta-CEL by iSatori Technologies are good products to try.

Fenugreek Seeds

What is it? Fenugreek seeds contain a high proportion (40 percent) of a soluble fiber known as mucilage. There is also a very interesting amino acid that is extracted from fenugreek seeds called 4-hydroxyisoleucine that may have an effect on insulin.

What does it do and how does it work? The fiber in fenugreek seeds forms a gelatinous structure (similar to guar gum) that may have effects on slowing the digestion and absorption of food from the intestines. Dietary fiber has been shown in many clinical studies to help control blood sugar and insulin levels (and even cause weight loss to occur). In terms of weight control, the soluble fiber in fenugreek seeds can reduce dietary fat absorption by binding to fatty acids as well as creating a sensation of "fullness" and reduced appetite—always a good thing when trying to control blood sugar levels! The amino acid 4-hydroxyisoleucine in fenugreek may stimulate insulin secretion (direct beta-cell stimulation) to regulate blood sugar.

What does the science say about it? Some studies indicate a beneficial effect of fenugreek in reducing blood glucose levels and improving glucose tolerance in patients with diabetes. Recent animal research (published in January 2006) showed that 4-hydroxyisoleucine lowers cholesterol, triglycerides, and free fatty acids. A 2005 study conducted at the University of Montana showed that this unique amino acid enhanced post-exercise glycogen resynthesis, which would be very helpful to exercising athletes because of the enhanced recovery and extra carbohydrates stored in muscle tissue. Other research confirms its effects as an insulin potentiator.

Dosage: For fenugreek, a typical dose is 300–500 mg daily of 4-hydroxy-isoleucine, preferably after a workout, and taken with carbohydrates and creatine.

Momordica Charantia

What is it? Momordica charantia (bitter melon extract) is a common plant/fruit that has a bitter taste (hence the name "bitter melon").

What does it do and how does it work? Bitter melon is yet another insulin mimicking and blood sugar regulating compound that has good research behind it. It lowers glucose concentration, improves glucose tolerance, and promotes glucose disposal into muscle tissue. What's interesting is that even after discontinuing this nutrient for a few weeks (after taking it for 30 days), bitter melon's effects can still be seen. According to some research, it works by improving insulin secretion by the beta cells of the pancreas or by possibly improving the action of insulin itself. This nutrient is especially useful to people who have late night cravings or have blood sugar imbalances.

What does the science say about it? This nutrient has been extensively studied in diabetics. In fact, one published review article states that it has been used in over 100 studies for diabetes and its complications. Research out of England also suggests it may have antioxidant activity, but that remains to be clearly validated. However, some of the studies on this nutrient showing benefits are not double-blind, placebo-controlled trials (the "gold standard" in research). Bitter melon does seem to have synergistic effects with other glucose-lowering agents.

Dosage: A typical dose is of bitter melon 100 mg, taken 1–3 times daily with meals (using a 4:1 standardized extract).

Remember, dosages on these supplements will vary according to your individual physiology, so it is best to contact your health-care provider to discuss supplementation based on your medical history.

Cortisol Blocking

A re you stressed out? Does your muscle soreness last for days after workouts in the gym? Is your mind less sharp than it used to be? Are your catabolic hormone (cortisol) levels through the roof? There are many sports supplements on the market today that promise dramatic results, from increasing lean muscle mass and releasing growth hormone to dropping body fat and many other things. Only some of these supplements are truly effective in producing measurable results on your physique and in the gym. One of these well-researched supplements is phosphatidylserine (PS). I know it's a mouthful, but after reading about this unique and powerful nutrient, it should be clear that this ingredient can enhance your bodybuilding efforts and should be considered an essential supplement, especially if you train hard.

Since this supplement is relatively unknown to many athletes, it is important to understand what it is and how it works. PS is a phospholipid, a type of fat found in every cell of the body that contains the mineral phosphorus, and the commercial supplement version is derived from either soy lecithin or bovine cerebral cortex. (Most of the versions on the market today are derived from soybeans due to the concern about "mad cow disease.") PS occurs naturally in some foods, such as green leafy vegetables and rice, but in very small, insignificant amounts. Supplementation is the only way to get enough PS to produce physiological results.

PS specifically contains a phosphatidyl molecule consisting of a head group containing phosphorus along with a chemical subgroup of serine. Phospholipids are vital to the proper function of cell membranes. In fact, phospholipids actually hold the molecules in the cell membranes together. PS imbedded into cell membranes can control many important functions, including movement of molecules in and out of the cell, taking cellular messages from the outside of the cell to its interior, and communication between cells. It can also help protect cell membranes from damage that can occur from intense training and free radicals.

PS is found in a high quantity in the brain and specifically in nerve cell membranes. Clinical research on PS dates back over twenty years but only recently have bodybuilders and other athletes realized all the benefits of this useful supplement.

Physiological Effects of Phosphatidylserine

Phosphatidylserine has been shown to have several positive effects in the body, including neurological enhancement, protection of cell membranes and boosting optimum cellular function, and cortisol suppression.

Neurological Enhancement

Most of the extensive research on phosphatidylserine is on its ability to improve brain function and memory. PS is highly concentrated in the brain, where it can help regulate the passing of impulses between nerve cells. It is also readily absorbed across the blood-brain barrier. In one study, subjects given 300 mg of PS daily for twelve weeks showed enhancement of memory and a greater ability to concentrate and focus as compared to the placebo group. Another study showed that individuals with moderate cognitive deterioration (some memory loss) had improved attention span, greater concentration, and short-term memory improvement by taking 300 mg of PS daily. Other studies also confirm these findings.

Cell Membrane Protection
and Optimum Cellular Function

Phosphatidylserine is found in cell membranes and can have a protective effect against cellular damage. Cellular damage can occur with age and even intense training, so having good levels of PS in the body is important. Optimal membrane levels of PS are important for sending signals into cells, including to secondary message systems. PS can also have an effect on the transport of key minerals in and out of cells, including calcium, sodium, potassium, and magnesium.

Cortisol Suppression

Research has shown that phosphatidylserine may be a powerful cortisol-suppressing agent. PS can lower ACTH (adrenocorticotrophin hormone) after exercise, which can help lower muscle breakdown secondary to exercise. According to several studies, PS supplementation can blunt cortisol release significantly secondary to stress. In fact, in one study, supplementation of PS at 800 mg daily reduced cortisol levels by 30 percent compared to a placebo following heavy resistance training.

The Effects of Cortisol in the Body

To truly appreciate these results with phosphatidylserine, it is essential to understand cortisol and its effects in the body. Cortisol is the primary glucocorticoid, a natural hormone produced by the adrenal glands. Cortisol is necessary to maintain important processes in times of prolonged stress. Most of its effects are not directly responsible for the initiation of metabolic or circulatory processes, but it is necessary for their full response.

The major catabolic effects of cortisol involve its facilitating the conversion of protein in muscles and connective tissue into glucose and glycogen (cortisol may increase liver glycogen). Gluconeogenesis involves both the increased degradation of protein already formed and the decreased synthesis of new protein. Cortisol can decrease the utilization of glucose by cells by directly inhibiting glucose transport into the cells and a cortisol excess may decrease insulin sensitivity. Cortisol also reduces the utilization of amino acids for protein formation in muscle cells. A cortisol excess can lead to a progressive loss of protein, muscle weakness and atrophy, and loss of bone mass through increased calcium excretion and less calcium absorption.

Recent research has shown that elevated cortisol levels increased protein breakdown by 5 percent to 20 percent. Even mild elevations in serum cortisol can increase plasma glucose concentration and protein catabolism within a few hours in healthy individuals. Cortisol levels rise with increasing time of intense exercise. Excess cortisol can also adversely affect tendon health. Cortisol causes a redistribution of body fat to occur through an unknown mechanism. Basically, the extremities lose fat and muscle while the trunk and face become fatter. Cortisol excess is linked to hypertension as well, because it causes sodium retention (which can make you appear bloated) and potassium excretion.

So, the real challenge becomes how can cortisol levels be controlled but not inhibited completely because of cortisol's necessary effects. One excellent way is to take a phosphatidylserine supplement regularly. With all the adverse effects of excess cortisol to muscle building, it is theorized that since PS blunts cortisol release, you can maximize your gains from training and optimize muscle recovery (cortisol delays muscle recovery) and muscle function by taking this supplement.

The way PS reduces cortisol levels is by suppressing hormones that control cortisol release, including ACTH and CRF (corticotropin-releasing factor). By using PS to reduce cortisol levels, you can increase the testosterone-cortisol ratio, which is a major determining factor of muscle anabolism in the body. It may be that since PS reduces cortisol levels, testosterone may work more efficiently in the body. So, PS can help reduce cortisol levels to lower muscle breakdown, but it does not cause a long-term detrimental suppression of cortisol.

By taking PS, athletes can recover from exercise much more quickly, thereby making faster gains in the gym. Interestingly, one of the mechanism's of action of anabolic steroids is also cortisol suppression, which is why athletes on anabolic steroids tend to recover much faster and have much less muscle soreness. The problem with anabolic steroids is that they block the corticosteroid receptor, which means that when individuals come off anabolic steroids, their cortisol levels soar and they experience muscle atrophy and a suppressed immune system. PS does not have the problem of cortisol receptor blockage and can be taken continuously in a safe and effective way.

Phosphatidylserine can play an important role in "overtraining syndrome." Overtraining can occur when there is a serious imbalance between training and proper recovery—not enough rest and optimal recovery from very intense training sessions. Overtraining has been shown to actually decrease performance, cause depression, promote injuries, and even lower immune health. In overtrained individuals, cortisol levels increase while testosterone levels decrease. PS can help speed up recovery and lower the negative effects from overtraining. It can also help repair damaged muscle cell membranes secondary to intense training. One study showed that athletes taking PS had much less muscle soreness and had a greater level of well-being even after just one week into the study. The group taking PS felt stronger and had greater energy levels.

Usage

The efficacious dose of phosphatidylserine ranges from 100 mg to 800 mg daily, depending on what you are using it for. For cognitive benefits and neurological function, as little as 100 mg daily may be effective, although 300 mg daily were used in many of the studies regarding this effect of PS. For athletic performance and bodybuilding purposes, a dose of 400 mg to 800 mg daily during periods of intense training can be effective. Remember, during times of intense training is when you can see and feel the effects of PS supplementation. The best times to take PS for cortisol suppression are right after training and/or thirty minutes before bedtime.

There is no reason to cycle PS as it has been shown to be safe even after long-term use. Some researchers believe PS may have blood-thinning properties, so it may be a good idea not to take PS with herbs like *Ginkgo biloba.* You should always consult a physician before taking PS if you have any medical conditions or are taking medications such as warfarin or other blood-thinning agents. Personally, PS has been one of the most effective supplements I have used. Its effects can be felt in as little as 1–2 weeks of use, especially if your workouts are intense. (And you know what they say, "Intensity builds immensity!") There are several high-quality phosphatidyl-serine supplements on the market, including Cort-Bloc from Muscle-Link, C3™ by EAS, and Serin-aid™ by Chemi Nutraceutical.

Hormone Modifiers

If you want to gain muscle, lose fat, or even boost exercise performance, it's all about hormones. Hormones are biologically active substances that regulate many key processes throughout the body. "Nothing can influence our body's shape more than our own hormones," says Karlis Ullis, M.D., a noted hormone expert and author of *The Hormone Revolution Weight Loss Plan.* "Hormones regulate weight, metabolism, how much muscle we have, food intake, and many other factors." This is true for both men and women. The key hormones affecting fat loss and muscle gain include growth hormone (GH) and IGF-1, testosterone (and estrogen), cortisol, insulin, and thyroid hormone.

Growth Hormone (GH)

Human growth hormone is the most abundant hormone of the pituitary gland, mainly released in pulses during sleep. GH has been shown to increase lean body mass, reduce body fat, increase energy, boost immune function, and even enhance sexual function. Normally, growth hormone secretion decreases with age.

Most of GH's powerful effects are due to its conversion in the liver to insulin-like growth factor type 1 (IGF-1). IGF-1 is what is actually measured in the blood test to determine GH levels in the body. In a 2002 study published in the *Journal of Nutrition*, men consuming soy protein isolate—40 grams (g) daily—had increased levels of serum IGF-1. Soy seems to stimulate GH levels when ingested, according to this study.

Obesity diminishes the release of GH and fasting helps increase it. Exercise is a potent stimulus for GH release.

145

Supplements That Boost Growth Hormone

- **Growth hormone–releasing peptides (GHRPs).** These oligopeptides, also known as secretagogues, have been shown to stimulate GH release. A relatively new study confirms the benefits of these secretagogues along with exercise; however, more research needs to be done. These products are quite expensive, but if you can afford them, they are worth trying, especially if you are over 40 years old (natural GH levels tend to decline after this age). Take GHRPs one hour before bedtime on an empty stomach. Some quality products in this category are GH-Stak by Muscle-Link and Secretagogue-One® by MHP.

- **L-Arginine.** This non-essential amino acid (sometimes considered "conditionally essential") has equivocal evidence that it can boost GH levels: some studies show little effect of L-arginine as a GH booster, while other studies show good results. Doses of 5–10 g before bedtime seem to work better (however, this amount may cause stomach discomfort in some people). Resverzene from ASR has a good dosage.

- **Alpha GPC.** Short for L-alpha-glycerylphosphorylcholine, this is an acetylcholine precursor derived from soy that has been shown in preliminary research to boost GH levels and increase neurological function. One plus is that smaller amounts, 150–400 milligrams (mg), seem to boost GH levels, which makes it more cost effective. A company called Chemi Nutraceutical produces Alpha GPC.

Insulin

Insulin is a peptide hormone that is released from the beta cells of the pancreas. It is released due to a rise in blood sugar levels, induced mainly by eating carbohydrates but to a lesser degree by some amino acids in protein foods. This hormone is primarily responsible for the direction of energy metabolism after eating. It can help transport key nutrients such as glucose and amino acids into muscle cells, but it can also cause fat storage to occur.

Nutritional Tips to Optimize Insulin

- **Eat low-glycemic meals that have little impact on blood sugar levels.** Mixed meals containing high-quality protein, complex carbohydrates, and essential fats are the key to stabilizing insulin levels.

- **Don't eat too many carbohydrates at night.** This can interfere with GH levels while you sleep, which is not good for optimal growth and recovery. Plus, this may lead to fat storage as metabolism is slower at night.

- **Spike blood sugar levels after a workout.** The post-workout period is a good time for consuming carbohydrates and protein to maximize recovery from training. A 3:1 or 4:1 ratio of carbohydrates to protein is recommended (for example, 60 g of simple carbs and 15 g of protein, preferably in liquid form).

Testosterone

Testosterone is a steroid hormone produced by the testes that promotes the development of male sex characteristics and regulates male reproductive function. It is called the most powerful muscle-building hormone because it does just that—builds muscle and strength fast. Testosterone increases muscle protein synthesis and net muscle protein balance, resulting in increased muscle mass. "Testosterone is one of the most effective hormones for burning fat in both men and women," states Dr. Ullis. Signs of low testosterone levels include low energy levels, muscle weakness, depression, and sexual dysfunction. Too much testosterone in males can convert into dihydrotestosterone (DHT), which can have adverse effects on the prostate gland plus cause hair loss, and estrogen, aromatization of which can lead to water retention, increased fat storage, and gynecomastia in males. It is important to measure both "free" testosterone (the active form) levels and estrogen levels to make sure there is not too much estrogen being produced. Estrogen can halt your muscle-building efforts.

Testosterone-Boosting Supplements

- **ZMA®.** ZMA is a highly specific and unique vitamin and mineral combination. There are certain minerals that have a positive impact on athletic performance as well as testosterone levels. ZMA is a special combination of zinc, magnesium, and vitamin B_6. Zinc is involved in the action of several hormones, including insulin, growth hormone, testosterone, and estrogen, and in more than 200 enzymatic reactions. Research has indicated that exercising individuals have a greater need for zinc and are more prone to a zinc deficiency. It is proven to increase testosterone levels in healthy subjects. A 1996 study showed that taking 30 mg of supplemental zinc daily by healthy men experiencing moderate zinc deficiency doubled their testosterone levels in a six-month time frame. Magnesium is involved in over 300 enzymatic reactions in the body, including glycolysis, the Krebs cycle, creatine phosphate formation, nucleic acid synthesis, amino acid activation, cardiac and smooth muscle contractability, cyclic AMP formation, and, most importantly for strength athletes, protein synthesis. Vitamin B_6 is also known as pyridoxine and has some major implications in protein synthesis. The coenzyme form of this vitamin is associated with a vast number of enzymes, the majority as part of amino acid metabolism. B_6 is necessary in glycogen catabolism to "unlock" carbohydrate energy and it has also been shown to diminish the actions of certain catabolic steroids, such as glucocorticoid hormones (cortisol). This can boost the testosterone-to-cortisol ratio, leading to positive muscle-building effects.

The zinc in this product is specifically formulated as zinc aspartate and zinc mono-L-methionine, which makes it more bioavailable. The magnesium is in a chelated form bound to aspartate, which increases its bioavailabity. Research with ZMA conducted on strength athletes shows that this combination of zinc, magnesium, and vitamin B_6 can increase total and free testosterone levels by 30 percent. A study published in *Medicine and Science in Sports and Exercise* showed that nightly supplementation with ZMA also increased strength and power. Taking one dose of ZMA about thirty minutes before bedtime is recommended.

- *Tribulus Terrestris.* This herb, used in Ayurvedic medicine, is also known as puncture vine and has been shown to boost testosterone levels naturally through a unique mechanism. It stimulates leutinizing hormone (LH) production from the anterior pituitary gland, which in turn stimulates testosterone production. Clinical studies have shown that *Tribulus* can enhance LH and free testosterone levels in healthy subjects by 70 percent and 40 percent, respectively. A Bulgarian study revealed that more than 200 men suffering from impotence—which is often caused by low testosterone levels—showed improved testosterone and LH levels as well as sperm production after the subjects supplemented with a preparation of *Tribulus terrestris*. The research also shows it to be very safe. It works at a divided dose of about 750–1,500 mg per day; good times to take it are first thing in the morning and one hour before a workout.

- **Fenugreek.** Fenugreek seeds contain active furostanol saponins, particularly diosgenin. Diosgenin has been proven to have various effects on cholesterol metabolism, specifically in lowering harmful LDL ("bad") cholesterol levels in animal studies. Furostanol saponins may exert effects on appetite stimulation and hormone release, which may support lean muscle mass and improved athletic performance. They have been implicated in positively impacting testosterone levels. TESTOFEN™ contains 50 percent steroidal saponins from defatted Fenugreek seeds. Taking 250 mg 2–3 times daily is a good dose.

- *Eurycoma Longifolia.* The root of this herb, commonly known as Tongkat Ali in Malaysia, has been used for centuries for treating fatigue, loss of sexual desire, and impotence. Plenty of research shows that it boosts sexual function as well as sexual desire. Several human studies also show that it may enhance testosterone levels through various mechanisms. The active ingredients include glycosaponins and eurypeptide compounds. Recent human clinical trials have shown that *Eurycoma* products LJ100™ from HP Ingredients and patented Longjax™ increase IGF-1 levels and modulate natural testosterone and cortisol levels. The bioactive eurypeptides seem to boost sex drive and function, in both men and women, by increasing testosterone levels and inhibiting sex hormone–binding globulin (SHBG), so that more free testosterone remains in the blood. Human clinical research conducted by Dr. Ismail Tambi, from the Specialist Reproduction Research Center, in Malaysia, has confirmed that LJ100 increases serum testosterone and DHEA levels and decreases SHBG levels significantly. *Eurycoma* holds promise for boosting testosterone levels and improving general health. Recommended amounts range from 100–300 mg in divided doses daily.

- 6-OXO®. 6-OXO (by ErgoPharm) is an estrogen blocker designed to help lower levels of this unwanted hormone in males. 6-OXO (4-etioallocholen-3,6, 17-trione) is a naturally occurring aromatase inhibitor, the enzyme responsible for converting excess testosterone into estrogen. Specifically, this means that it will irreversibly bind to the aromatase enzyme and deactivate it. Prolonged use of 6-OXO may result in a substantial reduction in the production of estrogen in the body, along with a coinciding upregulation of natural (testicular) testosterone production. This product is good for estrogen protection, but its one-dimensional effects make it an average testosterone booster. A good dose is 300 mg in divided doses daily.

Hormone Testing

Hormones can determine a lot about the success or failure of your fitness routine. There are two accurate ways to measure hormone levels—saliva and blood.

Saliva—The benefits of saliva testing are convenience and lower cost. Plus, saliva hormones are in their "free" or active states, so this allows for a very exact and accurate reading. Also, anyone can do this test without having to go through their doctor (except in California and New York). The downside is that thyroid hormone and IGF-1 levels are not usually available for testing with this method. A good source for saliva tests is ZRT Laboratory in Oregon (www.salivatest.com).

Blood—Blood testing is a more comprehensive and expensive way to test for hormones. The benefit is that you can test virtually anything using this method and it is more likely covered by insurance. However, it requires a visit to the doctor or a blood center. Your doctor can routinely perform these blood tests. If you want to do it yourself, try the Life Extension Foundation (www.lef.org) or go to one of their blood-drawing stations nationwide (for more informnation, call 1-800-208-3444). The recommended tests for both men and women are free testosterone, morning cortisol, estradiol, IGF-1, and free T3.

NORMAL RANGES FOR HORMONES		
	MEN	WOMEN
Testosterone*	50–200 pg/ml	20–50 pg/ml
Cortisol (morning)*	3.0–8.0 ng/ml	3.0–8.0 ng/ml
Estradiol*	0.5–1.5 pg/ml	1.5–5.0 pg/ml
IGF-1 (for GH)		
16–24 years old	182–780 ng/ml	182–780 ng/ml
25–39 years old	114–492 ng/ml	114–492 ng/ml
40–54 years old	90–360 ng/ml	90–360 ng/ml
Over 55 years old	71–290 ng/ml	71–290 ng/ml
Free T3	260–480 pg/ml	260–480 pg/ml

*From saliva testing.

P-450™ ([(S)-2,3-dihydro-5,7-dihydroxy-2-(3-hydroxy-4-methoxyphenyl)-4-H-1-benzopy-ran-4-one])

Hesperetin is an interesting citrus bio-flavonoid found primarily in oranges and lemons. The antioxidant properties of hesperetin are fairly well established. But a newly discovered, added benefit of this substance may be even more profound for weight trainers since hesperetin appears to be a potent anti-aromatase. Aromatase is the enzyme that is involved in the process through which hormones in the body are converted to estrogen. This is important because the conversion of testosterone to estrogen is thought to increase as we age (at least in males), and because increases in estrogen are linked to a whole host of unwanted side effects, like increased bodyfat, testicular shutdown, water retention, and in extreme cases, even gynecomastia (a "female-breast-like" appearance) or testicular cancer.

What's interesting is that no one has used this powerful anti-estrogen compound—until recently that is. Probably because hesperetin was virtually unknown until recent research indicated its potential positive effects for inhibiting estrogen and because it takes an immense amount of resources to learn how to extract such a compound from its natural source. Recently, however, hesperetin has been trademarked under the name P-450 and is sold commercially in a product called Isa-Test™ (www.isa-test.com). Since P-450 is a natural compound and it doesn't shutdown your body's natural production of testosterone, you can use it for as long as you'd like. A good dose is 200 mg at least once daily.

DHEA

Dehydroepiandrosterone (DHEA) is a natural hormone produced by the adrenal glands. It is considered the "mother" hormone, since it is a precursor to testosterone, progesterone, and estrogen production in the body. Some studies suggest it can boost testosterone levels but the proper and effective doses have always been in question. DHEA levels are known to decrease with age. DHEA converts into DHEA-S (sulfate) and androgens in the liver. It may be good for women and those looking for possible anti-aging effects, but its effects as a solid testosterone booster for most people under 40 are not that good.

Cortisol

Cortisol is the primary glucocorticoid and a natural hormone produced by the adrenal glands. Cortisol has many catabolic effects and can be detrimental to muscle building and fat loss. Cortisol excess can lead to a decrease in insulin sensitivity, progressive loss of protein, muscle weakness and atrophy, and loss of bone mass through increased calcium excretion and less calcium absorption. Recent research has shown that increased cortisol levels also increased protein breakdown by 5 to 20 percent. Cortisol levels rise with increasing time of intense exercise, especially weight training. Cortisol excess can also lead to hypertension because it causes sodium retention (which can make you appear bloated) and potassium excretion.

Bottom Line: Cortisol must be minimized, especially during sleep, to allow for maximum gains in muscle mass. Some signs of high cortisol levels include lethargy, muscle weakness, irregular sleep, depression, excess muscle soreness after workouts, and anxiety. Cortisol levels vary throughout the day, so it is important to have levels tested first thing in the morning for an accurate reading.

Cortisol-Suppressing Supplements

- **Phosphatidylserine (PS).** PS is a phospholipid (a type of fat found in every cell of the body that contains the mineral phosphorus) that research has shown to be a powerful cortisol-suppressing agent. PS supplementation can blunt cortisol release significantly secondary to stress. Taking 200–400 mg about 30 minutes before bedtime can speed recovery. Quality PS products are Cort-Bloc™ from MuscleLink and C3 by EAS.

- **Vitamin C.** This is a well-known antioxidant but it can also help reduce cortisol levels, according to some research. Taking 500–1,000 mg of vitamin C one hour before a weight-training workout can be helpful.

Thyroid Hormone

When people are trying to lose weight, they often experience a decrease in basal metabolic rate (BMR), the number of calories that you burn at rest. This is especially true after long periods of low-calorie dieting, use of stimulants (including ephedra and caffeine), and excessive amounts of physical activity (like too much cardio). The body seems to reduce metabolism after long periods of dieting as a defense mechanism, which may be why some people claim they cannot lose that last bit of fat no matter how much they exercise. The decrease in BMR is directly related to the level of thyroid hormone activity.

Thyroid hormone activity represents the levels of two hormones produced by the thyroid gland: thyroxine (T4) and triiodothyronine (T3). T4 is a low activity thyroid hormone and T3 (triiodothyronine) is a high-activity thyroid hormone. T4 converts into T3 in the liver. Thyroid hormones are very important for normal growth and development and maintaining metabolism and body weight. Thyroid hormones exert effects on thermogenesis and temperature regulation as well. They can enhance lipolysis (fat burning) in adipose (fat) tissue. When measuring thyroid hormones, it is important to test T3 levels, since this is the active form.

Supplements to Support Thyroid Hormone

- **Guggulsterones.** Guggulsterones (also known as guggulipid) comes from the plant *Commiphora mukul*, which has been around for hundreds of years as a component of Ayruvedic medicine. It can boost metabolism by increasing thyroid hormone levels (both T4 and T3). There are several studies that have shown the effects of guggulipid as a fat-reducing compound. A good dose is 25 mg of active guggulsterones (after standardization) taken three times daily. Try MX-LS7 by iSatori Technologies or Lipo-6® by Nutrex Research.

- **Phosphates.** These are mineral compounds that contain phosphorus and may help boost metabolism and possibly exercise performance. According to a 1996 study published in the *Journal of Physiology and Pharmacology*, a combination of calcium, potassium, and sodium phosphates were shown to increase resting metabolic rate (RMR) in overweight women who were on a low-calorie diet. The researchers concluded that phosphates may play a role in the peripheral metabolism of thyroid hormones, specifically by preventing a decrease in T3 output. A good dose is 1 g of phosphates taken one hour prior to exercise. Try Phosphate Edge™ by FSI Nutrition.

Joint Health
and Repair

I f you think osteoarthritis is something that afflicts only aging baby boomers and nursing-home residents, you should talk with former world-class gymnast Bart Conner. Conner, who more than twenty years ago took home two Olympic gold medals and was considered one of America's top all-around athletes, today can hardly take out the garbage. He was diagnosed with osteoarthritis in his mid-20s. Or talk with professional tennis star Martina Hingis, who, at twenty-one, had to take a hiatus from the sport due to severe pain in her left ankle, knee, and hip. Her doctors say she already may be showing signs of osteoarthritis in her injured joints.

You can even talk to any bodybuilder who has been training for many years and they'll tell you about their joint problems. A growing number of strength athletes in their 20s and 30s are discovering firsthand that osteoarthritis isn't just a problem for grandma or grandpa anymore. A study from the University of Washington supports many other studies that show athletes, especially resistance-training athletes who hit it hard day in and day out, are at high risk for the debilitating joint disease.

At present, doctors believe that osteoarthritis afflicts more than 20 million Americans. By 2020, that number is expected to reach 40 million. Indeed, some researchers think that we're headed for a full-blown epidemic of degenerative joint disease. Results of a 2002 nationwide survey from the U.S. Centers for Disease Control and Prevention (CDC) showed that 69.9 million adults—roughly one-third of the U.S. adult population—suffer from arthritis or chronic joint pain symptoms.

Joint Disease Can Bring Your Training to a "Grinding" Halt

Osteoarthritis is a degenerative joint condition characterized by the erosion of the cartilage at the ends of the bones. Cartilage is the shock absorber of the joint and without it joint problems can occur. Due to wear and tear on the joints, the once tough and slippery cartilage that separates the bones may become soft, frayed, and thinned—it basically wears through like an old sock, leaving rough boney surfaces to grind on one another every time the joint moves.

Scientists have also recently identified a host of other things that can cause cartilage degradation and osteoarthritis. Weak quadriceps muscles can stress the knee joint. Eroding cartilage can cause painful bone spurs, but changes in bone structure can actually erode cartilage as well. When

Joint and Other Injuries

Injuries can be detrimental to a weight training or athletic training program. However, there are many ways around injuries that can allow you to continue experiencing good results from your program. Remember, if you have a serious injury, consult your physician before starting or continuing any exercise program.

Knee—Knee injuries are common in older individuals and, if they occurred in the gym, are usually caused by improper technique. If the injury occurred outside of the gym, then proper treatment depends on the severity of the injury. If you have tendinitis (mainly in the patella tendon) in the joint, then a multi-ingredient glucosamine-based formula may be very helpful to enhance fluid in the joints, repair cartilage, and decrease inflammation. Obviously, if you have a serious injury that affects your ability to walk, you need to see a doctor immediately—preferably a specialist such as an orthopedic surgeon.

Many individuals who have minor knee injuries generally have overtrained their quadricep muscles without effectively strengthening their hamstrings and calves. It is very important to train all areas of the legs equally to prevent any imbalances that may occur. Avoiding exercises like deep barbell squats; replacing them with leg press exercises may be beneficial.

cartilage erodes, certain immune cells come in and help get rid of the tissue but they also seem to attack healthy joint tissue, which can cause inflammation. Finally, certain genes play a role in predetermining cartilage status.

Left untreated and unchecked, this can become very debilitating for the hard-training athlete. Chronic osteoarthritis has ended the careers of numerous athletes, including future Hall of Fame quarterback and two-time Super Bowl Champion John Elway, formerly of the Denver Broncos. Many of us close to John say he still had the desire to play another year or two, but his joints just couldn't take the punishment, so he had to retire.

Treatment and Preventative Options

Along with an estimated 5 million other Americans, Elway takes two nutrients called glucosamine and chondroitin sulfate, which taken together or sepa-

Remember not to lock out the knees on a leg press movement and keep toes pointed outwards to prevent stress on the knee joint.

Shoulders—Shoulder injuries are also fairly common in the gym. Many involve the muscles of the rotator cuff, including the infrasupinatus and teres minor muscles. It is important again to see a doctor if any of these injuries are serious. Avoiding exercises like deep behind-the-neck barbell presses and barbell bench presses may help. If the rotator cuff is damaged, then ice for twenty minutes and heat for twenty minutes can be beneficial. Again, a multi-ingredient glucosamine-based formula can help repair and enhance the recovery process. Using a lighter weight and performing movements that do not cause any pain in the affected area are also highly recommended.

Lower Back—This is probably the most common problem among weight trainers and exercising individuals. One of the most common things that causes this imbalance to occur is weak abdominal and oblique muscles. It is very important to strengthen the abdominal and oblique muscles from every angle to solidify the torso. Avoiding exercises like deep squats with improper form, bent over barbell rows, deadlifts using a jerking motion, seated cable rows, barbell curls swinging the weights, and other movements using improper form may be beneficial. The ice-and-heat method mentioned earlier can help with lower back pain. As always, a multi-ingredient glucosamine-based formula can aid in speeding up the road to recovery from an injury.

rately are now America's top-selling joint supplements. These two substances, naturally found around cartilage cells, have been shown in clinical trials to be effective for people with osteoarthritis by alleviating symptoms and perhaps even repairing battered joints. Let's take a closer look at these and a few of the other top joint products and the research surrounding their use.

Glucosamine

What is it? Glucosamine, a naturally occurring compound comprised of glucose and a derivative of the amino acid glutamine, is an integral part of all forms of connective tissue in your body: cartilage, ligaments, and tendons. It can even serve as a precursor to synovial (joint) fluid by stimulating something called glycosaminoglycans (GAGs). Most of the glucosamine on the market is commercially derived from shellfish, so if you have an allergy, it may be best to avoid this nutrient.

What does it do and how does it work? While it isn't clear exactly how glucosamine works, scientists suggest the long-term effects with glucosamine could be due to its positive effects on cartilage regeneration, including stimulation of anabolic activities such as the synthesis of compounds called "proteoglycans," which ultimately results in improved joint function. It also seems to enhance the joint (synovial) fluid, helping lubricate the joint.

What does the science say about it? Double-blind studies have shown that glucosamine may be more effective than ibuprofen for relieving the pain and inflammation of osteoarthritis. And although the pain-relieving effects of glucosamine don't seem to be as immediate as with analgesics, the important point is that glucosamine may work quite differently to relieve pain, according to some research, by actually regenerating cartilage and thus repairing the arthritic damage.

In a 2001 study in *The Lancet,* a team of researchers in Liege, Belgium, tested glucosamine on 212 people with osteoarthritis in their knees. Subjects were given either a placebo or 1,500 milligrams (mg) of glucosamine daily over three years. By comparing a series of patients' knee x-rays, researchers reported that by the end of the study patients taking glucosamine experienced a 20 to 25 percent improvement of their symptoms, while the placebo group experienced a slight worsening of symptoms. The x-rays showed that joint spaces in the untreated patients had narrowed by an average of 0.31 millimeters, compared to no significant joint-space loss among those who supplemented with glucosamine. Earlier studies have also shown promising findings, but each called for long-term trials to confirm the results. According to the Council for Responsible Nutrition (CRN), this rigorously conducted study reported in *The Lancet* answers the call.

Dosage: The typical dose of glucosamine is 500 mg taken three times daily. Look for glucosamine sulfate or glucosamine HCl—these are the best absorbed and most readily available forms.

Chondroitin Sulfate

What is it? Chondroitin sulfate is a component of a biological polymer (polymers are substances with a high molecular weight) that is derived from tissue, such as ligaments, tendons, and cartilage.

What does it do and how does it work? Chondroitin sulfate is popularly used because some research shows it may strengthen and add flexibility to the protein filaments that compose connective tissues. Research also shows the nutrient may reduce inflammation and inhibit the production of enzymes that weaken connective tissue by attacking tendons and ligaments. It may therefore be effective for use in rehabilitating and even preventing some types of injuries, such as torn ligaments and tendons or damaged cartilage.

What does the science say about it? In an earlier study on osteoarthritis patients, a group of French researchers found that oral chondroitin sulfate may be an effective pain-relieving agent. From cartilage samples taken at the end of three months of therapy, researchers have also found that chondroitin users appeared to experience less tissue damage.

Research has shown that chondroitin may be even more effective when combined with glucosamine. In fact, the combination may have synergistic effects. In a 2000 review of the scientific literature on glucosamine and chondroitin published in the *Journal of the American Medical Association* (*JAMA*), researchers from The Arthritis Center at the Boston University School of Medicine noted that glucosamine and chondroitin preparations for osteoarthritis symptoms demonstrated "moderate to large effects."

Another review of the glucosamine and chondroitin research published in 2001 in the *Bulletin on the Rheumatic Diseases* noted that glucosamine's and chondroitin's disease-modifying effects in osteoarthritis were supported by the preliminary data. Newly published research (2005) from the Czech Republic confirms that a glucosamine/chondroitin combination can relieve pain and improve range of the joint motion as well as have mild anti-inflammatory effects.

Dosage: A typical dose of chondroitin sulfate is 400 mg three times daily.

Nexrutine™

What is it? Nexrutine is a plant extract developed from the phellodendron tree (*Phellodendron amurense*).

What does it do and how does it work? Nexrutine seems to inhibit the gene expression of an enzyme called COX-2, which is responsible for producing the sensation of pain in joints and muscles. Nexrutine may actually help decrease muscle and joint soreness without the negative effects of NSAIDs (nonsteroidal anti-inflammatory drugs) such as ibuprofen.

What does the science say about it? Several studies have shown that this nutrient may work not only to suppress inflammation but also to block pain at the source. Recent research shows NSAIDs may interfere with muscle growth and recovery and perhaps even increase the breakdown of cartilage in joints of people suffering from joint problems. Nexrutine may be a good alternative.

Dosage: A typical dose of Nexrutine is 250 mg three times daily.

Type II Collagen

What is it? Collagen is derived from the cartilage and bones of chickens and cows. It contains chondroitin sulfate, hyaluronic acid (HA), and glucosamine sulfate.

What does it do and how does it work? Type II collagen's mechanism of action seems to be in its components—chondroitin sulfate, hyaluronic acid, and glucosamine sulfate. These components support proteoglycans and glycosaminoglycans (GAGs) in the joint matrix, thereby increasing synovial fluid and supporting cartilage synthesis. This can enhance a joint's shock absorption capabilities as well as lower the chance for deterioration. In rheumatoid arthritis, natural collagen within the joints is gradually destroyed, apparently because an immune system attack floods the area with tissue-destroying white blood cells. Researchers believe type II collagen may stimulate a natural mechanism in the body that tones down the white blood cell attack on the patient's own collagen.

What does the science say about it? Type II collagen has been shown in a number of studies to help ease symptoms of certain arthritic conditions, primarily those from rheumatoid arthritis but also osteoarthritis. However, other research has shown only small and inconsistent benefits from oral supplementation with type II collagen. In a 1993 study of 60 patients, published in *Science*, researchers from Boston's Beth Israel Hospital found that 80 percent of the subjects experienced decreased joint swelling and tenderness after three months of supplementation compared to only 13 percent in the placebo group. Four patients in the collagen group had complete remission of the disease. In a 2000 study review of collagen for osteoarthritis and osteoporosis, the researchers found a high level of safety for hydrolyzed (heat treated) collagen and recommended it as an attractive agent for long-term use in these chronic disorders.

Dosage: Typically, take 1,000 mg of collagen in two divided doses daily. A good form of collagen, in liquid form, is CH Alpha™. Contained in convenient ready-to-drink vials, this form is more bioavailable than pills. Another good product is BioCell Collagen II® from BioCell Technology.

MSM (Methyl-Sulfonyl-Methane)

What is it? MSM is a metabolite of DMSO (dimethylsulfoxide), which is used to relieve joint and muscle pain and is generally applied topically.

What does it do and how does it work? MSM is a major sulfur donor. Sulfur is very important for the maintenance of connective tissue. Sulfur is involved in many metabolic pathways and plays an important structural role in amino acid metabolism. Sulfur is required for proper synthesis and maintenance of connective tissues such as skin, nails, tendons, and cartilage.

What does the science say about it? According to a study in the *Alternative Medicine Review Journal*, MSM is a volatile component in the sulfur cycle and increases in serum sulfate explain many of MSM's therapeutic effects.

Dosage: Typically take 2 g of MSM daily in two divided doses. People with any allergies should consult their physician.

CMO (Cetyl Myristoleate)

What is it? CMO is an oil or fatty acid–based nutrient. It is usually derived from a natural bovine source.

What does it do and how does it work? CMO seems to act as a joint lubricant and anti-inflammatory agent for osteoarthritis and rheumatoid arthritis.

What does the science say about it? Several studies show that CMO enhanced mobility in patients with osteoarthritis. A 2004 study published in the *Journal of Rheumatology* showed greater unilateral balance with CMO. Another study published in the same journal in 2002 also stated that "CMO may be an alternative to the use of nonsteroidal anti-inflammatory drugs (NSAIDs) for the treatment of osteoarthritis."

Dosage: A typical dose of CMO is 500 mg three times daily.

White Willow Bark

What is it? White willow bark is a natural form of salicylic acid (an aspirin-like compound). It comes from the bark of the white willow tree.

What does it do and how does it work? White willow bark may offer the joint pain–relieving and anti-inflammatory effects of aspirin without being hard on the stomach or interfering with muscle recovery.

What does the science say about it? According to a Canadian review article published in 2006, two trial of *Salix alba* (white willow bark) found some evidence that 120 mg or 240 mg of standardized salicin taken daily were better than placebo for short-term improvements in pain. An additional trial demonstrated white willow bark's relative equivalence to 12.5 mg per day of rofecoxib (Vioxx). So, it may have modest drug-like effects.

Dosage: Typically take 60–100 mg of salicin (after standardization) from white willow bark in two divided doses daily.

Supportive Vitamins and Minerals

Vitamin C plays an important role in collagen synthesis and also has antioxidant effects, which may lower the risk of free radical damage of the joints. Manganese, silica, and boron also play important co-factor roles in optimum joint and bone function.

LEVEL 4

Supplemental Matters

Supplement
Timing

W hat you do before, during, and after your workout can make all the difference in terms of gaining strength and muscle mass. It's easy to build muscle, right? Train hard, eat smart, and you're there. We all wish it was that simple. "Intensity builds immensity" and so you train super hard, but what if you aren't making the gains you are capable of? Maximizing pre-workout, workout, and post-workout nutrition can lead to much greater gains in muscle mass and strength, so much so that everyone at the gym may wonder what "you're on." There are advanced nutritional and supplementation strategies employed by the highest caliber athletes that can create astronomical gains in your physique. It's time to shed some light on this sometimes confusing subject and set the record straight. Please keep in mind that there are supplements that combine many of these ingredients into one product. All the best nutrients are mentioned for each specific time, but it is not necessary to take them all to have good effects. You can take some or a majority of them and still make gains.

Pre-Workout

Everyone wants to maximize their workout to create a better body. Have you noticed that when you are not focused or excited about working out, it can have a detrimental effect on your physique development? Did you know there are nutritional and supplementation strategies to almost guarantee a great workout every time?

Before we get to that, let's look at the energy systems of the body and what they use for fuel during exercise. Weight training mainly uses the phosphocreatine (PCr) energy system, which supplies the body with energy for activity lasting less than 8 seconds (explosive and short-duration activity is dependent on this system). Creatine and phosphate supplementation can maximize this energy system. For activities lasting longer than 8 seconds and up to 30 seconds, the body uses a little of the PCr system but mainly uses the glycolytic energy system (anaerobic glycolysis primarily). This system requires carbohydrate from food sources or from stored carbohydrate energy (glycogen) in the liver and muscle tissue. The body uses anaerobic and aerobic glycolysis for activity lasting greater than 30 seconds and up to about 2 minutes, again requiring carbohydrate. Finally, activity lasting greater than 2 minutes mainly uses the oxidative energy system, which requires fat. Now that the energy systems have been defined, let's examine the goals of pre-workout nutrition to maximize exercise performance.

Goals

There are several metabolic events that are absolutely necessary to achieve before a workout. Optimizing the availability of carbohydrates, protein, and fluid (hydration) are essential. Consuming carbohydrates before training can increase glycogen stores and provide energy during the workout. It is crucial to consume a carbohydrate-rich and protein meal about two hours before training. Complex carbohydrates like sweet potatoes or brown rice are preferred at this time to further enhance glycogen storage and stabilize blood sugar levels to prevent a mid-workout crash, which can occur if simple sugars are taken before a workout. Carbohydrates are critical for muscle contraction and delaying muscle fatigue, especially during stressful exercise.

Protein and essential amino acid (EAA) availability is vital before a workout as well to help lower muscle breakdown secondary to weight training. Amino acid supplementation has a positive effect on protein synthesis. The idea is to create an anabolic environment for muscle growth—increases in protein synthesis while lowering protein breakdown. One of the signals for stimulating protein synthesis is the availability and extracellular concentrations of essential amino acids. In a recent study in the *Canadian Journal of Applied Physiology,* the researchers found that a mixture of essential amino acids and carbohydrates stimulates muscle protein synthesis more effectively when taken before rather than after exercise. Based on this study, taking 20 grams (g) of protein, mainly from whey protein isolate (containing about 50 percent EAAs and 25 percent branched-chain amino acids, which can help recovery, increase protein synthesis, and support exercise performance), and 20 g of carbohydrates about thirty minutes before training can have a positive effect on muscle growth. Other research indicates that consuming protein and carbohydrates before heavy resistance exercise can boost insulin-like growth factor type 1 (IGF-1) and growth hormone levels. Boosting levels of these two hormones may create a favorable environment for muscle growth.

Hydration is also very important before a workout (it's important during and after your workout too). Water is the best thing for hydration before a workout. Try to consume at least 16 ounces within one hour before training. Some research demonstrates that dehydrating a muscle by as little as 3 percent can cause a 12 percent loss of strength—not good when you're trying to push up heavy weights in the gym or competing on the field.

Maximizing testosterone levels and "priming" the body to lower cortisol levels during and after the workout are two key factors to consider before a workout. Since testosterone is the muscle-building hormone, boosting natural levels before training can have a positive effect on your workout. Cortisol, the catabolic hormone involved in muscle breakdown, needs to be minimized during and after training, but pre-workout nutrition has to initiate this effect. Carbohydrate intake and the subsequent insulin response can lower cortisol levels.

Free radicals (oxidative compounds that can damage muscle cells and have been implicated as causes of many diseases) need to be suppressed when weight training or competing in sports. It has been proven that strenuous physical exercise causes a significant rise in free radicals, as much as 100- to 200-fold during exercise. This can overwhelm the body and delay recovery from a workout. It may also cause greater amounts of infection and sickness in some athletes. Antioxidants help quench free radicals and can provide many beneficial effects against exercise-related oxidative tissue damage. It is essential to take a mixture of antioxidants to fight free radicals and boost immune function. This is especially key if your diet is deficient and your training is intense. Some great immune boosters and antioxidants include vitamins C and E, beta-carotene, alpha-lipoic acid, and NAC (N-acetyl-cysteine).

Sometimes we all need a "pick me up" before a workout, which is where stimulants come into play. Stimulating the nervous system and enhancing neurotransmitter output can boost mental focus and clarity. After all, so much of athletics and working out is mental. Neurotransmitter fatigue or even burnout can lead to "bonking" during the workout. Some stimulants can even boost performance.

Pre-Workout Supplement Strategy

- **Caffeine.** Caffeine seems to stimulate skeletal muscle directly through calcium release and by increasing cyclic AMP levels, which is a secondary messenger system in cells that can increase hormone usage and have other ergogenic benefits. Caffeine can also spare muscle glycogen levels during exercise, delaying muscle fatigue and time to exhaustion and allowing you to get a few more reps at the gym. Optimum dosage is 200 mg of caffeine (in pill form) taken about one hour prior to exercise. If you have any medical conditions, consult a physician before using this powerful supplement.

- **Tyrosine.** This amino acid can enhance neurotransmitter output and may promote greater mental focus and performance, especially under stressful conditions. A dose of 1–2 grams (g) of tyrosine one hour before a workout may work well.

- *Ginkgo biloba.* This herb has been clinically proven to increase blood flow to the brain and enhance neurological function, which may increase focus while training. A specific extract of this herb (EGB-761) can actually lower cortisol levels as well. A typical dose is 60–120 milligrams (mg) of *Ginkgo biloba* (standardized to 24 percent glycosides and 6 percent terpene lactones) about an hour before training.

- **Phosphatidylserine (PS).** This phospholipid is a powerful cortisol-suppressing agent. Several clinical studies show the cortisol-lowering effects of PS, especially secondary to weight training. Take 400 mg of PS one hour before training to lower cortisol levels during and after training. An added bonus is the brain-boosting effects of PS, which includes protecting brain cells from damage that can occur over time. And it also seems to enhance mental acuity and concentration, which is always useful.

- *Tribulus terrestris.* This herb can help boost natural testosterone levels by stimulating LH (leutinizing hormone) and "turning on" testosterone production. Taking 500 mg of *Tribulus terrestris* one hour before training may help.

- **ZMA.** This supplement is a special combination of zinc and magnesium along with vitamin B$_6$ for energy and can help enhance exercise performance. One study shows that ZMA can boost natural testosterone levels and strength in athletes. In fact, magnesium supplementation by itself has been shown to increase strength and protein synthesis. Take the recommended dosage on the bottle—usually four pills.

- **Antioxidants.** Antioxidants can suppress damaging free radicals. Vitamin C is one of the best antioxidants. It has been shown to lower oxidative stress caused by exercise and blunt cortisol levels as well. Vitamin C also seems to decrease post-workout inflammation when it is taken before a workout. Other studies have shown the benefits of combining vitamins C and E along with beta-carotene to decrease oxidative stress secondary to exercise in advanced athletes. Alpha-lipoic acid and N-acetylcysteine (NAC) can also be used effectively to support immune function. Recommended doses vary, but 500–1,000 mg of vitamin C, 200–400 international units (IU) of vitamin E, and 32 mg of beta-carotene can be very effective taken ninety minutes before a workout.

- **Phosphates.** Potassium phosphate may enhance recovery after exercise. Phosphates may also delay fatigue by buffering lactic acid and they can also help store creatine better in muscle cells, which would lead to greater energy levels inside muscle cells. Although not essential, it may be a good idea to take 1 g of phosphates one hour before training.

- **L-Carnitine.** This amino acid may enhance fat utilization when taken prior to exercise. Some research also shows that L-carnitine L-tartrate (a special form) can assist significantly in recovery from hard training. This supplement is not a necessity, but try taking 1 g about thirty minutes before a workout.

- **Arginine.** This "conditionally essential" amino acid helps regulate protein synthesis, nitric oxide production, and immune function. It can even release growth hormone when taken in high doses. Take 2–5 g within thirty minutes before a workout.

During Workout

The important thing during the workout is to keep energy levels higher and delay muscle fatigue, especially by buffering lactic acid. Taking special drinks during a workout can help you keep going longer and stronger.

Goals

It is important to maximize energy reserves, which means consuming simple sugars to provide quick energy for the workout. Buffering lactic acid, thereby delaying fatigue, is always a good thing and lowering cortisol levels is helpful too. Minimizing free radicals and maintaining a proper electrolyte balance (which may reduce the chance of cramping) is a key component as well. Many of these goals can be accomplished by consuming the more advanced sports drinks on the market. Eating an energy bar during the workout instead of drinking a sports beverage is not good because eating solid food requires water for digestion, which can pull water out of muscle tissues. It is also absorbed much more slowly than a liquid drink and may even cause stomach discomfort in some people. Moral of the story—no nutrition bars during exercise.

During Workout Supplement Strategy

- **Sports Drink.** A sports drink that contains mainly dextrose (glucose), maltodextrin, and some fructose with a 5 to 7 percent total carbohydrate concentration is a good choice. Carbohydrate ingestion and the insulin release that follows can help keep cortisol levels low throughout the workout and even into recovery. Carbohydrate drinks can lower physiological stress and inflammation secondary to exercise and they can elevate exercise performance. However, too much fructose in sports drinks can cause an upset stomach. One important factor to look for in sports drinks is osmolality, which measures the concentration of particles in solution. A sports drink should have an osmolality of 250–300 mOsm/kg. Normal body fluids have an osmolality of about 275–300 mOsm/kg, so a solution that exceeds this level becomes hypertonic (a cell that is hypertonic has a greater concentration of water than its environment; osmosis transports water out of the cell causing cellular dehydration). This can negatively affect water balance.

- **BCAAs, Electrolytes, and Antioxidants.** Look for the electrolytes sodium, potassium, phosphate, and magnesium in a good sports drink. The branched-chain amino acids (BCAAs) leucine, isoleucine, and valine may help delay muscle fatigue and prolong exercise, especially in the heat, when taken during a workout. Antioxidants that stop free radicals are always good during training, when free radicals are being produced at a high rate. Try to get all of these nutrients in liquid form for optimal absorption during a workout.

Post-Workout

The post-workout period is by far the most important time for anyone trying to build a better body. What you do in the 2–4 hours following a workout can determine what kind of gains you will make in your physique and if you will get stronger or not. The greatest nutrient uptake occurs after a hard weight-training workout—you've depleted nutrients and now the body is ready to take them back. Some experts even recommend consuming 50 percent of your total daily calories within 2–4 hours after a hard workout.

There are several reasons why nutrient absorption is heightened significantly post-workout. First, insulin sensitivity is greatest after a workout and this helps transport nutrients like glucose, amino acids, and creatine into muscle cells. Insulin can also cause fat storage with excess calories. When insulin sensitivity is increased, most of the glucose and amino acids transported by insulin go right to the muscle cells and fat storage is minimized. Glucose taken up rapidly by the muscle cells following exercise can then cause glycogen production and greater carbohydrate storage in muscle tissue. This is essential for creating an anabolic environment for growth.

Research has clearly demonstrated that muscle glycogen synthesis is twice as rapid if carbohydrates are consumed immediately after exercise as opposed to waiting for a few hours. Research has also found that combining protein with carbohydrate right after a workout can further enhance glycogen synthesis, even more than with just carbohydrates alone. In fact, a protein and carbohydrate drink after a workout can maximize insulin levels for several hours following weight training. The addition of the amino acid L-arginine to a carbohydrate supplement post-exercise increased the availability of glucose for muscle glycogen storage.

One of the reasons glycogen synthesis is enhanced after a workout is because the enzyme responsible for glycogen production—glycogen synthase—is up-regulated and glucose transporters in muscle cells are also active. The protein synthesis machinery of muscle cells is also activated in a greater way. That is why consuming protein post-workout can help enhance protein synthesis, muscle repair, and amino acid availability.

Goals

The key post-workout goal is to increase muscle anabolism (increase protein synthesis while decreasing or minimizing muscle breakdown). Lowering cortisol, replenishing glycogen stores, providing amino acids and carbohydrates in the optimum 4:1 ratio (or at least a 3:1 ratio) for maximum glycogen replenishment, and increasing cell volume to create a greater anabolic environment in the cell are all very important after a workout. It is also critical to maximize insulin levels to drive nutrients into muscle cells. Hydration with water at this time is important to help enhance cell volumization and transport nutrients in the body. Taking a post-workout recovery drink is essential to proper workout recovery and muscle building.

Post-Workout Supplement Strategy

- **Protein/Carbohydrate Drink.** This drink should be taken immediately after exercise and consist of a 4:1 ratio of carbohydrates to protein (about 100 g carbs and 25 g proteins). The protein should be from high-quality whey protein isolate, while the carbohydrates should consist of simple sugars with a high glycemic index (dextrose, glucose, and maltodextrin). Whey protein isolate contains a high dose of BCAAs and essential amino acids and is readily absorbed by the body. Remember, timing is everything and in the post-workout period it is important to get amino acids into muscle tissue as soon as possible. Many research studies validate the use of a post-workout recovery drink. A 2001 study published in the *Journal of Physiology* found that intake of an oral protein supplement after resistance exercise was important for the development skeletal muscle. Carbohydrate supplementation right after a workout and one hour afterwards can decrease muscle breakdown and create a more positive body protein balance.

    Those of you trying to lose weight who think a post-workout drink with carbohydrates is not for you, think again. New research indicates that consuming a protein/carbohydrate drink immediately after a workout can increase resting metabolic rate (RMR), which can increase metabolism and help with fat loss. So, make sure you have a post-workout drink ready every time. Consume it right after a workout; then, one hour after training, have some more protein and carbohydrates (a meal replacement powder would be great at this time). Then, 2.5 hours after training, have a whole-food source of protein along with some complex carbohydrates and fibrous vegetables.

- **Creatine.** Research has clearly demonstrated that creatine can boost muscle mass, strength, and muscle size. Taking creatine after a workout is better than before or during training, contrary to popular belief. It is better absorbed and stored after weight training. Since creatine transport is insulin-dependent and insulin levels are elevated after a workout, creatine can have greater uptake into muscle tissue, where it is stored until it is used. Creatine also has a cell volumizing (anabolic) effect, which is always good after a workout. Take 5 g of creatine and mix it with your protein/carbohydrate drink right after a workout.

- **Glutamine.** Glutamine is the most abundant amino acid in muscle tissue. Supplemental glutamine can help promote cell volumization (draw more water inside muscle cells, creating a more anabolic environment for growth), increase protein synthesis, and decrease the breakdown of proteins, while partially determining the rate of protein turnover in muscles. Glutamine peptide is better absorbed than free-form glutamine (due to peptide transport systems in the digestive tract) and it is also more stable in solution. Speed of nutrient uptake is essential after training. Wheat protein hydrolysate (a common source for glutamine peptide) has been shown to increase glycogen synthesis. According to research from the Swedish University of Agricultural Sciences, glutamine concentration is 10 percent higher in type II muscle fibers compared to type I fibers. Type II muscle fibers have a large disposition for growth and are used mainly in weight training. After exercise, the same researchers showed a 45 percent decrease in glutamine in both fiber types—hence the need for supplementation. A good dose is 5–10 g of glutamine or glutamine peptide consumed right after a workout, and then 5 g more ingested ninety minutes after training.

- **BCAAs.** These special amino acids have been shown to act directly in potentiating protein synthesis, lowering muscle breakdown, sparing protein, and enhancing overall recovery. A good whey protein isolate supplement has plenty of BCAAs. Supplementation with higher doses of BCAAs may also be useful.

- **Taurine.** This is the second most abundant amino acid in muscle tissue.

It can cause cell volumization, has insulin-mimicking properties, and can help support protein synthesis. A good dose of taurine is 2–4 g right after a workout.

- *Rhodiola rosea.* This adaptogenic herb has been shown to reduce stress and enhance the recovery process secondary to exercise. Taking 100 mg of *Rhodiola rosea* after a workout may be beneficial.

- **Chromium Polynicotinate.** This mineral has been shown to aid in weight loss, but it also enhances insulin sensitivity. Taking 400 micrograms (mcg) after a workout can further enhance nutrient uptake into muscle tissue and allow insulin to work more effectively.

- **Alpha-Lipoic Acid.** This compound is both a fat- and water-soluble antioxidant and it can support nutrient transport by mimicking insulin. Taking 100 mg of alpha-lipoic acid after a workout can be helpful.

- **Fenugreek.** There is a very interesting amino acid that is extracted from fenugreek seeds called 4-hydroxyisoleucine. This ingredient may stimulate insulin secretion (direct beta-cell stimulation) and help control blood sugar levels. Again, this can allow for greater transport of key nutrients like creatine, amino acids, and glucose into muscle tissue.

- **Vitamins C and E.** These antioxidants can help scavenge free radicals lurking around after a workout. Free radicals can delay the recovery process and damage muscle cells. Taking 500 mg of vitamin C and 400 IU of vitamin E after a workout is a good idea and can speed up recovery and enhance overall health.

The importance of proper pre-workout, during workout, and post-workout nutrition and supplementation cannot be overstated. Keep in mind that there are supplements from various companies that can fit the bill for some of these goals. Now, it's time to implement these advanced, research-based strategies to maximize your muscle-building potential.

Integrated Sports-Specific Supplement Programs

More and more professional athletes are discovering the benefits of using nutrition supplements. We've designed supplement programs for dozens of Olympic and professional athletes. For the most part, the supplements these world-class athletes use to help build muscle, reduce body fat, and improve athletic performance are the ones you can benefit from as well. Many athletes have experienced unprecedented success using supplement programs.

Make no mistake, these aren't garden-variety supplement programs—they are very specific, not to mention very expensive if you decide use *all* the recommended nutrients. Of course, using every one of the nutrients recommended here is *not* necessary. Remember, start with a good foundation (Level 1) and work up. Building a good foundation—making sure you're fending off deficiencies common to athletes by getting the essential nutrients needed—maximizes your potential for enjoying the full performance-enhancing effects of the Level 2 and Level 3 nutrients. (Please note that the dosages listed below are for the average 180-pound male and need to be adjusted for anyone else.) Many of these ingredients can also be found combined in single products.

BASEBALL

Goals

- Increase bat/pitching speed, mental focus, and quickness
- Increase power and lean muscle mass
- Reduce the risk of muscle cramps, pulls, and strains

- Strengthen joints and connective tissue

Integrated Supplementation

Level 1 (Foundation) Nutrients: MRPs, protein bars, essential fatty acids (EFAs), vitamins and minerals (including additional magnesium, potassium, phosphates, calcium, and iron).

Level 2 (Essential) Supplements: Glucosamine, creatine, glutamine, taurine, and antioxidants (including N-acetylcysteine, vitamins C and E, and beta-carotene).

Level 3 (Performance) Supplements: Carbohydrate/electrolyte–containing sports drink, type II collagen, MSM, caffeine, L-tyrosine, *Rhodiola rosea*, DMAE, *Ginkgo biloba*, and phosphatidylserine.

The Program

MRPs: Take 1–2 packets/servings daily in place of meals, preferably mixed with water. Take one after a game or practice. Eat-Smart® Nutrition Shake, Myoplex RTD, and Labrada's Lean Body are good options.

Protein bars: Take 1–2 bars daily, preferably as a snack one to two hours before a game or practice.

EFAs: Take 2 tablespoons of flaxseed oil or a blend such as Udo's Choice Perfected Oil Blend daily; take 1 tablespoon with your first and second meals.

Vitamins and minerals: Take a good multivitamin/multimineral blend as a safety net daily.

Glucosamine: Take 500 milligrams (mg) three times daily with meals.

Creatine: See the chapter on creatine for special loading instructions. Take 5 grams (g) daily, 2.5 g before and 2.5 g after a hard workout, practice, or game. Try 3-XL or Phosphagen Elite.

Glutamine: Take 5–10 g daily, one dose after a game, workout, or practice and then another dose forty-five minutes before bedtime.

Taurine: Take 2–4 g before a practice or game and then another 2–4 g afterward. You may even take it during the game or practice to help lower the incidence of cramping and enhance recovery.

Antioxidants: Take a good antioxidant formula daily (such as Noxidant from SciVation).

Carbohydrate/electrolyte–containing sports drink: A carbohydrate sports drink that contains mainly dextrose (glucose), maltodextrin, and some fructose (at a 5 to 7 percent carbohydrate concentration) along with key minerals is a good choice. Endurathon from EAS and Accelerade from Pacific Health Labs are recommended choices.

Type II collagen: Take 500 mg 2–3 times daily with meals to strengthen connective tissue. A good product is CH Alpha.

Methylsulfonylmethane (MSM): Take 500 mg 2–3 times daily to support healthy joints.

Caffeine: This stimulant may delay fatigue and enhance sports performance. Take 200–400 mg of pure caffeine 30–45 minutes before a game. Pure caffeine has been shown to be more effective than coffee.

L-Tyrosine: This amino acid may enhance neurotransmitter output and promote greater mental focus and performance, especially under stressful conditions. A dose of 1–2 g one hour before a game or practice may work well. A good combination of caffeine and L-tyrosine can be found in Energize.

Rhodiola rosea: Take 100 mg of this herb three times a day. Take 200 mg one hour before a game or practice and then 100 mg after a game or practice.

DMAE: DMAE (2-dimethylaminoethanol) is a natural chemical produced in the brain that boosts levels of the neurotransmitter acetylcholine. This may improve mood, mental clarity, focus, and short-term memory. Take 100–300 mg one hour before a game.

Ginkgo biloba: This herb may increase blood flow to the brain and enhance mental focus. Take 100–200 mg of ginkgo (standardized to 24 percent glycosides and 6 percent terpenes) one hour before a game or practice.

Phosphatidylserine (PS): Take 400 mg of PS after a hard workout, game, or practice and another 400 mg of PS forty-five minutes before bedtime.

Before Game/Practice

Protein bar: 1–2 hours before a game
Creatine: 2.5 g
Taurine: 2 g
Antioxidants: 1 serving
Rhodiola rosea: 200 mg

Caffeine: 200 mg
Gingko biloba: 100 mg
L-Tyrosine: 1 g
DMAE: 100 mg

During Game/Practice

Carbohydrate/electrolyte–containing sports drink and 3 g of taurine

L-Tyrosine: 500 mg

After Game/Practice

MRP: 1 serving

Rhodiola rosea: 100 mg

L-Glutamine: 5 g

Taurine: 2 g

Creatine: 2.5 g

HMB: 1 g

Phosphatidylserine: 400 mg

MSM: 500 mg

Type II collagen: 500 mg

FOOTBALL

Goals

- Increase size, strength, and speed

- Reduce the risk for injuries by strengthening joints

- Reduce the risk of muscle cramps, pulls, and strains

Integrated Supplementation

Level 1 (Foundation) Nutrients: MRPs, whey protein, vitamins and minerals, and EFAs.

Level 2 (Essential) Supplements: Glucosamine, creatine, glutamine, taurine, HMB (beta-hydroxy-beta-methylbutyrate), and antioxidants.

Level 3 (Performance) Supplements: Post-workout/game recovery drink, carbohydrate-containing sports drink, type II collagen, *Rhodiola rosea,* Alpha-GPC, and phosphatidylserine.

The Program

MRPs: Take 1–3 daily in place of meals, preferably mixed with skim milk. Eat-Smart® Nutrition Shake, Myoplex RTD, and Lean Body are good options.

Vitamins and minerals: Take a good multivitamin/multimineral blend (such as Opti-Pack from Super Nutrition) as a safety net daily.

EFAs: Take 2 tablespoons of flaxseed oil (or a blend such as Udo's Choice Perfected Oil daily); 1 tablespoon with the first and second meals.

Glucosamine: Take 500 mg three times daily with meals.

Creatine: See the chapter on creatine for special loading instructions. Take 5 g daily, 2.5 g before and 2.5 g after a hard workout, practice, or game.

Glutamine: Take 5–10 g daily, one dose after a game, workout, or practice, and then another dose 45 minutes before bedtime. EAS or MHP are good sources.

Taurine: Take 2–4 g before a practice or game and then another 2–4 g afterward. You can even take it during the game or practice.

HMB: Take 3–4 g daily in divided doses.

Antioxidants: Take a good antioxidant formula daily (like Noxidant from Sci-Vation).

Post-workout recovery drink: Take 1 serving after a hard practice or game. Good ones include Endurox R4, Surge from Biotest, and 3-XL from iSatori Technologies.

Carbohydrate/electrolyte–containing sports drink: A carbohydrate sports drink that contains mainly dextrose (glucose), maltodextrin, and some fructose (at a 5 percent–7 percent carbohydrate concentration) along with key minerals is a good choice. Endurathon from EAS and Accelerade from Pacific Health Labs are recommended choices.

Type II collagen: Take 500 mg 2–3 times daily with meals to strengthen connective tissue. CH Alpha is a good choice.

Rhodiola rosea: Take 100 mg three times a day; take 200 mg one hour before a game or practice and then 100 mg afterward.

Alpha-GPC: Take 300 mg of Alpha-GPC 45 minutes before bedtime daily.

Phosphatidylserine (PS): Take 400 mg of PS after a hard workout, game, or practice and another 400 mg of PS forty-five minutes before bedtime.

Before Game/Practice

Creatine: 2.5 g
Taurine: 3 g
HMB: 1 g

Antioxidants: 1 serving
Rhodiola rosea: 200 mg

During Game/Practice

Carbohydrate/electrolyte–containing sports drink and 1 g of taurine
Whey protein isolate: 10 g

After Game/Practice

Post-workout recovery drink
Rhodiola rosea: 100 mg
L-Glutamine: 5 g
Taurine: 2 g

Creatine: 2.5 g
HMB: 1 g
Phosphatidylserine: 400 mg

GOLF

Goals

- Increase mental focus and swing power
- Strengthen joints and connective tissue
- Stay well-hydrated on course

Integrated Supplementation

Level 1 (Foundation) Nutrients: MRPs, protein bars, EFAs, vitamins, and minerals.

Level 2 (Essential) Supplements: Glucosamine, creatine, and antioxidants (including NAC, vitamins C and E, and beta-carotene).

Level 3 (Performance) Supplements: Carbohydrate/electrolyte–containing sports drink, type II collagen, MSM, L-tyrosine, DMAE, *Ginkgo biloba*, and phosphatidylserine.

The Program

MRPs: Take 1–2 packets/servings daily in place of meals, preferably mixed with water. Take one after a round on the course. Eat-Smart® Nutrition Shake, Myoplex RTD, and Labrada's Lean Body are good options.

Protein bars: Take 1–2 bars (containing 25–30 g of carbohydrates and 20–25 g of protein) daily, preferably as a snack one to two hours before a round.

EFAs: Take 1–2 tablespoons of flaxseed oil (or a blend like Udo's Choice Perfected Oil Blend) daily; 1 tablespoon with the first and second meals.

Vitamins and minerals: Take a good multivitamin/multi-mineral blend daily (like Opti-Pack from Super Nutrition) as a safety net.

Glucosamine: Take 500 mg three times daily with meals.

Creatine: Take 2 g before a round and 2 g afterward.

Antioxidants: Take a good antioxidant formula (like Noxidant from Sci-Vation) daily.

Carbohydrate/electrolyte–containing sports drink: A carbohydrate sports drink that contains mainly dextrose (glucose), maltodextrin, and some fructose (at a 5 percent–7 percent carbohydrate concentration) along with key minerals is a good choice. CytoVol RTD from EAS and Accelerade from Pacific Health Labs are recommended choices.

Type II collagen: Take 500 mg two to three times daily with meals to strengthen connective tissue. CH Alpha is a good choice.

Methylsulfonylmethane (MSM): Take 500 mg two to three times daily to support healthy joints.

L-Tyrosine: This amino acid can enhance neurotransmitter output and may promote greater mental focus and performance especially under stressful conditions. A dose of 1–2 g one hour before a round may work well. Energize from iSatori Technologies or L-Tyrosine from Kaizen are good choices.

DMAE: DMAE (2-dimethylaminoethanol) is a natural chemical produced in the brain that boosts levels of the neurotransmitter acetylcholine. This can improve mood, mental clarity, focus, and short-term memory. Take 100–300 mg one hour before a round.

Ginkgo biloba: This herb increases blood flow to the brain and may enhance mental focus. Take 100–200 mg of ginkgo (standardized to 24 percent glycosides and 6 percent terpenes) one hour before a round.

Phosphatidylserine (PS): Take 200 mg of PS forty-five minutes before a round.

Before Round (on the course)

Protein bar: 1–2 hours before start
Creatine: 2 g
Antioxidants: 1 serving
Ginkgo biloba: 100 mg

L-Tyrosine: 1 g
DMAE: 100 mg
Phosphatidylserine: 200 mg

During Round

Carbohydrate/electrolyte–containing sports drink
L-Tyrosine: 500–1,000 mg

After Round

MRP: 1 serving   MSM: 500 mg
Creatine: 2 g   Type II collagen: 500 mg

SOCCER

Goals

- Increase speed and quickness

- Enhance endurance and reduce muscle fatigue

- Reduce the risk of muscle cramps, pulls, and strains

Integrated Supplementation

Level 1 (Foundation) Nutrients: MRPs, protein bars, vitamins, and minerals (including additional magnesium, potassium, phosphates, calcium, and iron).

Level 2 (Essential) Supplements: Glucosamine, creatine, glutamine, taurine, HMB, antioxidants (including NAC), vitamins C and E, and beta-carotene.

Level 3 (Performance) Supplements: Post-workout/game recovery drink, carbohydrate/electrolyte–containing sports drink, caffeine, glycerol, BCAAs (branched-chain amino acids), *Rhodiola rosea*, and phosphatidylserine (PS).

The Program

MRPs: Take 1–2 daily in place of meals, preferably mixed with water. Eat-Smart® Nutrition Shake, Myoplex RTD, and Lean Body are good options.

Vitamins and minerals: Take a good multivitamin/multimineral blend (like Opti-Pack from Super Nutrition) as a safety net daily. The formula should provide at least 750 mg of magnesium, 1,200 mg of calcium, a 3:1 ratio of potassium to sodium, 1 g of phosphates, and 18 mg of iron daily.

Protein bars: Take 1–2 bars daily, preferably as a snack one to two hours before a game or practice.

Glucosamine: Take 500 mg three times daily with meals.

Creatine: See the chapter on creatine for special loading instructions. Take 5 g daily, 2.5 g before and then 2.5 g after a hard workout, practice, or a game. Try 3-XL or Phosphagen Elite.

Glutamine: Take 5–10 g daily, one dose after a game, workout, or practice, and then another dose 45 minutes before bedtime.

Taurine: Take 2–4 g before a practice or game and then another 2–4 g afterward. You can even take it during the game or practice. This may help lower the incidence of cramping and enhance recovery.

Antioxidants: Take a good antioxidant formula daily (like Noxidant from Sci-Vation).

Post-workout recovery drink: Take 1 serving after a hard practice or game. Good ones include Endurox R4, Surge from Biotest, and RecoverX from MuscleLink.

Carbohydrate/electrolyte–containing sports drink: A carbohydrate sports drink that contains mainly dextrose (glucose), maltodextrin, and some fructose (at a 5 to 7 percent carbohydrate concentration) along with key minerals is a good choice. Endurathon from EAS and Accelerade from Pacific Health Labs are recommended choices.

Caffeine: Caffeine may delay fatigue and enhance sports performance. Take 200–400 mg of pure caffeine 30–45 minutes before a game. (Pure caffeine has been shown to be more effective than coffee.)

BCAAs (branched-chain amino acids): The BCAAs leucine, isoleucine, and valine may help delay muscle fatigue and prolong exercise, especially in the heat, when taken during a workout. Take 5 g of BCAAs during a game or practice and 2–3 g afterward.

Rhodiola rosea: Take 100 mg of this herb three times a day. Take 200 mg one hour before a game or practice and then 100 mg afterward.

Phosphatidylserine (PS): Take 400 mg of PS after a hard workout, game, or practice, and another 400 mg of PS forty-five minutes before bedtime.

Before Game/Practice

Creatine: 2.5 g
Taurine: 3 g
Antioxidants: 1 serving
Rhodiola rosea: 200 mg
Caffeine: 200 mg

During Game/Practice

Carbohydrate/electrolyte–containing sports drink and 2 g of taurine
BCAAs: 5 g

After Game/Practice

Post-workout recovery drink
Rhodiola rosea: 100 mg
L-Glutamine: 5 g

Taurine: 2 g
Creatine: 2.5 g
Phosphatidylserine: 400 mg

TENNIS

Goals

- Increase power and speed
- Reduce mental fatigue
- Reduce the risk for injuries by strengthening joints
- Reduce the risk of muscle cramps, pulls, and strains

Integrated Supplementation

Level 1 (Foundation) Nutrients: MRPs, vitamins and minerals (including extra magnesium and potassium), and EFAs.

Level 2 (Essential) Supplements: Glucosamine, creatine, glutamine, taurine, and antioxidants.

Level 3 (Performance) Supplements: Carbohydrate/electrolyte–containing sports drink, caffeine, L-tyrosine, *Rhodiola rosea*, and *Siberian ginseng*.

The Program

MRPs: Take 1–2 daily in place of meals, preferably mixed with cold water. Eat-Smart® Nutrition Shake, Myoplex RTD, and Labrada's Lean Body are good options.

Vitamins and minerals: Take a good multivitamin/multimineral blend (like Opti-Pack from Super Nutrition) as a safety net daily.

Magnesium: Take 400 mg (as magnesium citrate or glycinate) one hour before a match or practice.

Potassium: Take 300 mg (as potassium citrate) one hour before a match or practice.

EFAs: Take 1 tablespoon of flaxseed oil (or a blend like Udo's Choice Perfected Oil Blend) daily with your first meal.

Glucosamine: Take 500 mg three times daily with meals.

Creatine: Take 4 g daily, 2 g before and then 2 g after a hard practice or match. Try 3-XL or Phosphagen Elite.

Glutamine: Take 5 g daily, one dose after a match or practice.

Taurine: Take 2–4 g before a practice or match and then another 2–4 g afterward. You can even take a dose during the match to help lower the chances of cramping.

Antioxidants: Take a good antioxidant formula (like Noxidant from SciVation) daily.

Carbohydrate/electrolyte–containing sports drink: A carbohydrate sports drink that contains mainly dextrose (glucose), maltodextrin, and some fructose (at a 5 to 7 percent carbohydrate concentration) along with key minerals is the way to go. Endurathon from EAS and Accelerade from Pacific Health Labs are recommended choices.

Caffeine: Take 200 mg of caffeine thirty minutes prior to a match or practice. An additional 100 mg can be taken during the match.

L-Tyrosine: Take 1–2 g thirty minutes before a match or practice to enhance mental focus. Energize from iSatori Technologies or L-Tyrosine from Kaizen are good formulas.

Rhodiola rosea: Take 100 mg of this herb three times a day. Take 200 mg one hour before a match or practice and then 100 mg afterward.

Siberian ginseng: Take 250 mg one hour before a match or practice.

Before Match/Practice

Magnesium: 400 mg

Potassium: 300 mg

Creatine: 2 g

Taurine: 3 g

Antioxidants: 1 serving

Caffeine: 200 mg

L-Tyrosine: 1 g

Rhodiola rosea: 200 mg

Siberian ginseng: 250 mg

During Match/Practice

Carbohydrate/electrolyte–containing sports drink and 1 g of taurine, plus an additional 100 mg of caffeine and 1 g of L-tyrosine.

After Match/Practice

Rhodiola rosea: 100 mg

Creatine: 2 g

L-glutamine: 5 g   MRP: 1 serving
Taurine: 2 g

TRACK AND FIELD

(This obviously depends on what event you participate in, but we'll stick to the majority of the running events.)

Goals

• Increase speed and quickness

• Enhance endurance and reduce muscle fatigue

• Reduce the risk of muscle cramps, pulls, and strains

Integrated Supplementation

Level 1 (Foundation) Nutrients: MRPs, vitamins, and minerals (including additional magnesium, potassium, phosphates, calcium, and iron).

Level 2 (Essential) Supplements: Glucosamine, creatine, glutamine, taurine, antioxidants (including NAC), vitamins C and E, and beta-carotene.

Level 3 (Performance) Supplements: Post-workout/event recovery drink, carbohydrate/electrolyte–containing sports drink, caffeine, glycerol (for endurance running events), BCAAs (branched-chain amino acids), *Rhodiola rosea*, and phosphatidylserine (PS).

The Program

MRPs: Take 1–2 daily in place of meals, preferably mixed with water. Eat-Smart® Nutrition Shake, Myoplex RTD, and Lean Body are good options.

Vitamins and minerals: Take a good multivitamin/multimineral blend (like Opti-Pak from Super Nutrition) as a safety net daily. The formula should provide at least 750 mg of magnesium, 1,200 mg of calcium, a 3:1 ratio of potassium to sodium, 1 g of phosphates, and 18 mg of iron daily.

Glucosamine: Take 500 mg three times daily with meals.

Creatine: See the chapter on creatine for special loading instructions. Take 5 g daily, 2.5 g before and then 2.5 g after a hard workout, practice, or event. Try 3-XL or Phosphagen Elite.

Glutamine: Take 5–10 g daily, one dose after a race, workout, or practice, and then another dose forty-five minutes before bedtime.

Taurine: Take 2–4 g before a practice or event and then another 2–4 g afterward. You can even take it during the game or practice. This may help lower the incidence of cramping and enhance recovery.

Antioxidants: Take a good antioxidant formula daily (like Noxidant from Sci-Vation).

Post-workout recovery drink: Take one serving after a hard practice or event. Good ones include Endurox R4, Surge from Biotest, and Recover-X from MuscleLink.

Carbohydrate/electrolyte–containing sports drink: A carbohydrate sports drink that contains mainly dextrose (glucose), maltodextrin, and some fructose (at a 5 to 7 percent carbohydrate concentration) along with key minerals is a good choice. Endurathon from EAS and Accelerade from Pacific Health Labs are recommended choices.

Caffeine: Caffeine may delay fatigue and enhance sports performance. Take 200–400 mg of pure caffeine 30–45 minutes before an event. (Pure caffeine has been shown to be more effective than coffee.)

Glycerol: To enhance hyper-hydration, take 3–4 tablespoons of glycerol mixed with 16–24 ounces of water one hour before a long running event or practice.

BCAAs (branched-chain amino acids): The BCAAs leucine, isoleucine, and valine may help delay muscle fatigue and prolong exercise, especially in the heat, when taken during a workout. Take 5 g of BCAAs during a game or practice and 2–3 g afterward.

Rhodiola rosea: Take 100 mg of this herb three times a day. Take 200 mg one hour before a event or practice and then 100 mg afterward.

Phosphatidylserine (PS): Take 400 mg of PS after a hard workout, event, or practice, and another 400 mg of PS forty-five minutes before bedtime.

Before Event/Practice

Creatine: 2.5 g

Taurine: 3 g

Antioxidants: 1 serving

Rhodiola rosea: 200 mg

Caffeine: 200 mg

Glycerol: 40–60 g with 16–24 ounces of water

During Event/Practice

Carbohydrate/electrolyte–containing sports drink and 2 g of taurine
BCAAs: 5 g

After Event/Practice

Post-workout recovery drink   Creatine: 2.5 g
Rhodiola rosea: 100 mg   Phosphatidylserine: 400 mg
L-Glutamine: 5 g   Taurine: 2 g

"BULKING UP"/GAINING MUSCLE MASS

Integrated Supplementation

Level 1 (Foundation) Nutrients: Weight gainer, EFAs, and vitamins, and minerals (including additional magnesium, potassium, phosphates, calcium, and iron).

Level 2 (Essential) Supplements: Creatine, glutamine, antioxidants (including NAC)

Level 3 (Performance) Supplements: Post-workout recovery drink, L-arginine, beta-alanine, 6-OXO, and *Tribulus terrestris.*

The Program

Weight gainer: Take 2–3 recommended servings of a product like True Mass from BSN, CytoGainer from Cytosport, and Mass-Tech from MuscleTech.

EFAs: Take 2 tablespoons of flaxseed oil or a blend such as Udo's Choice Perfected Oil Blend daily; take 1 tablespoon with your first and second meals.

Vitamins and minerals: Take a good multivitamin/multimineral blend as a safety net daily. A good product is Opti-Pack from Super Nutrition.

Creatine: See the chapter on creatine for special loading instructions. Take 10 g daily, 5 g before and 5 g after a hard workout. Take 5 grams first thing in the morning on non-training days. Try 3-XL or Phosphagen Elite.

Glutamine: Take 5–10 g daily, one dose after a workout, and then another dose forty-five minutes before bedtime.

Antioxidants: Take a good antioxidant formula (such as Noxidant from Sci-Vation) daily. Take one recommended dose in the morning and one dose before training.

Post-workout recovery drink: Take one serving after a hard practice or game. Good ones include Endurox R4, Surge from Biotest, and Recov-erX from MuscleLink.

L-arginine: Take 5 g (1 tsp) before a workout and 5 g one hour prior to bed-time.

Beta-alanine: Take 1.6 g before a workout and 1.6 g right after a workout. Two recommended products are Red Dragon™ by Muscle-Link, and H-Blocker from iSatori Technologies.

6-OXO: Take 100 mg in the morning and 100 mg before a workout.

Tribulus terrestris: Take 500 mg before exercise and 500 mg before bedtime. Isa-Test™ and Vitrix™ are good formulas.

"CUTTING UP"/LOSING BODY FAT

Integrated Supplementation

Level 1 (Foundation) Nutrients: MRPs, protein bars, and vitamins, and minerals (including additional magnesium, potassium, phosphates, calcium, and iron).

Level 2 (Essential) Supplements: Glutamine, branched-chain amino acids, and antioxidants (including NAC).

Level 3 (Performance) Supplements: Thermogenic supplement, gugguls-terones, alpha-lipoic acid, CLA, and phosphatidylserine

The Program

MRPs: Take 1–2 daily in place of meals, preferably mixed with water. Eat-Smart® Nutrition Shake, Myoplex RTD, and Lean Body are good options.

Vitamins and minerals: Take a good multivitamin/multimineral blend (like Opti-Pack from Super Nutrition) as a safety net daily. The formula should provide at least 750 mg of magnesium, 1,200 mg of calcium, a 3:1 ratio of potassium to sodium, 1 g of phosphates, and 18 mg of iron daily.

Protein bars: Take one bar daily, preferably as a snack between meals.

Glutamine: Take 5–10 g daily, one dose after a workout and then another dose forty-five minutes before bedtime.

Antioxidants: Take a good antioxidant formula daily (like Noxidant from Sci-Vation).

BCAAs (branched-chain amino acids): The BCAAs leucine, isoleucine, and valine may help delay muscle fatigue and prolong exercise, especially in the heat, when taken during a workout. They may also help reduce abdominal fat. Take 5 g of BCAAs after a workout (for advanced lifters, an additional 5 g before the workout may also help).

Thermogenic fat burner: Take one serving before cardio or a workout and an additional serving with lunch. Start these slow and work up to the recommended dosage. If you have any medical issues, please consult a doctor before using. Good choices are MX-LS7 or Lean System 7 for men, and Curvelle™ or Fareinheit™ for women.

Guggulsterones: 25 mg three times daily with meals.

Alpha-lipoic acid: 100 mg three times daily with meals, preferably one dose before and after a workout.

CLA: 1 g three times daily with meals. Look for the Clarinol or Tonalin brand names to make sure you are getting quality CLA.

Phosphatidylserine (PS): Take 400 mg of PS after a hard workout and another 400 mg of PS forty-five minutes before bedtime.

REDUCE MUSCLE SORENESS AND OPTIMIZE RECOVERY

Integrated Supplementation

Level 1 (Foundation) Nutrients: MRPs, vitamins, and minerals (including additional magnesium, potassium, phosphates, calcium, and iron).

Level 2 (Essential) Supplements: L-glutamine, branched-chain amino acids, taurine, glucosamine, methylsulfonylmethane (MSM), and antioxidants (including NAC). Recoverzene from ASR contains many of these nutrients.

Level 3 (Performance) Supplements: Alpha-lipoic acid, beta-alanine, *Rhodiola rosea,* and phosphatidylserine

The Program

MRPs: Take 1–2 daily in place of meals, preferably mixed with water. Eat-Smart® Nutrition Shake, Myoplex RTD, and Labrada's Lean Body are good options.

Vitamins and minerals: Take a good multivitamin/multimineral blend (like Opti-Pack from Super Nutrition) as a safety net daily. The formula should provide at least 750 mg of magnesium, 1,200 mg of calcium, a 3:1 ratio of potassium to sodium, 1 g of phosphates, and 18 mg of iron daily.

Glutamine: Take 5–10 g daily, one dose after a workout and then another dose forty-five minutes before bedtime.

Glucosamine: Take 500 mg three times daily with meals.

MSM: Take 500 mg 2–3 times daily.

Antioxidants: Take a good antioxidant formula daily (like Noxidant from Sci-Vation).

BCAAs (branched-chain amino acids): The BCAAs leucine, isoleucine, and valine may help delay muscle fatigue and prolong exercise, especially in the heat, when taken during a workout. They may also help reduce abdominal fat. Take 5 g of BCAAs after a workout (for advanced lifters, an additional 5 g before the workout may also help).

Taurine: Take 2 g before a workout and 2 g after a workout.

Alpha-lipoic acid: 100 mg three times daily with meals, preferably one dose before and after a workout.

Beta-alanine: Take 1.6 g before and after a workout. Two recommended products are Red Dragon™ by Muscle-Link, and H-Blocker from iSatori Technologies.

Rhodiola rosea: 100 mg three times daily—one dose before and after a workout.

Phosphatidylserine (PS): Take 400 mg of PS after a hard workout and another 400 mg of PS forty-five minutes before bedtime.

INCREASE AEROBIC PERFORMANCE

Integrated Supplementation

Level 1 (Foundation) Nutrients: MRPs, vitamins, and minerals (including additional magnesium, potassium, phosphates, calcium, and iron).

Level 2 (Essential) Supplements: Creatine, L-glutamine, taurine, BCAAs (branched-chain amino acids, and antioxidants (including NAC), vitamins C and E, and beta-carotene.

Level 3 (Performance) Supplements: Citrulline malate, carbohydrate/electrolyte–containing sports drink, caffeine, and *Rhodiola rosea.*

The Program

MRPs: Take 1–2 packets daily in place of meals, preferably mixed with water. Eat-Smart® Nutrition Shake, Myoplex RTD, and Labrada's Lean Body are good options.

Vitamins and minerals: Take a good multivitamin/multimineral blend (like Opti-Pack from Super Nutrition) as a safety net daily. The formula should provide at least 750 mg of magnesium, 1,200 mg of calcium, a 3:1 ratio of potassium to sodium, 1 g of phosphates, and 18 mg of iron daily.

Creatine: See the chapter on creatine for special loading instructions. Take 5 g daily, 2.5 g before and then 2.5 g after a hard workout. Try 3-XL or Phosphagen Elite.

Glutamine: Take 5–10 g daily, one dose after a workout and then another dose 45 minutes before bedtime.

Taurine: Take 2 g before and after a workout. This may help lower the incidence of cramping and enhance recovery.

BCAAs (branched-chain amino acids): The BCAAs leucine, isoleucine, and valine may help delay muscle fatigue and prolong exercise, especially in the heat, when taken during a workout. Take 5 g of BCAAs during a workout and 2–3 g afterward.

Antioxidants: Take a good antioxidant formula daily (like Noxidant from SciVation).

Carbohydrate/electrolyte–containing sports drink: A carbohydrate sports drink that contains mainly dextrose (glucose), maltodextrin, and some fructose (at a 5 to 7 percent carbohydrate concentration) along with key minerals is a good choice. Endurathon from EAS and Accelerade from Pacific Health Labs are recommended choices. Take during exercise.

Citrulline malate: Take 3 g before a workout. A good product is H-Blocker from iSatori Technologies.

Caffeine: Caffeine may delay fatigue and enhance sports performance. Take 200–400 mg of pure caffeine 30–45 minutes before a workout. (Pure caffeine has been shown to be more effective than coffee.)

Rhodiola rosea: Take 100 mg of this herb three times a day. Take 200 mg one hour before a workout and then 100 mg afterward.

Delivery Systems for Supplements

The form in which you take a supplement can make a big difference in the effectiveness of your nutritional program. There are several key issues that supplement forms or delivery systems have to address:

- Efficiently delivering nutrients to key places like muscles

- Allowing nutrients to be readily and quickly absorbed into the blood-stream

- Decreasing stomach discomfort associated with some nutrients

- Allowing nutrients with a short half-life (they get in and out of the body fast) to stay in the body longer to prolong their effects

- Protecting sensitive and fragile nutrients from being destroyed by stomach acid when taken orally

Timed (sustained or controlled) release technology has become popular because it prevents a large "dumping" of nutrients in the body by more slowly releasing nutrients over time. This dumping effect can minimize the effectiveness of some ingredients. Many delivery systems for supplements actually come from the pharmaceutical industry. Using these pharmaceutical delivery systems, key nutrients can be maximized and consumers basically get more bang for their buck by enhancing absorption and uptake of nutrients. There's nothing worse than buying a product and only utilizing 5 percent of it.

Tips to Remember

One other thing to keep in mind is that some nutrients are better absorbed when taken with certain foods or other nutrients, while other supplements are better absorbed when taken on an empty stomach. For example, fat-soluble vitamins like D and E are better absorbed when taken with some sort of fat. Caffeine can be better utilized and its effects enhanced if it is taken with naringin (from grapefruit). The absorption of yohimbe can also be enhanced if taken with some fat-containing food, due to its low bioavailability. Creatine delivery to muscle cells is enhanced when combined with simple carbohydrates that cause an insulin response. It can also be enhanced with sodium and a mixture of protein and simple carbohydrates too. It is important to remember not to take certain supplements that need to be quickly absorbed with fiber-containing foods, as this may slow absorption.

Types of Supplement Delivery Systems

Capsules

Capsules are probably the most widely used delivery system for supplements. Most gelatin-based capsules are dissolved in around 20 minutes. There are veggie caps (non-meat derivative) and halal/kosher caps now available. There are varying sizes and many nutrients can be delivered this way.

Tablets

These are unique in that they can dissolve within minutes or hours, depending on the coating, the fiber-based fillers in them, and their specified pH (acid/alkaline balance). Tablet-making technology has advanced quite a bit. They can now even be made to dissolve in certain areas of the digestive system, such as the first part of the small intestine where many nutrients are more effectively absorbed. If timed-release technology or controlled-release technology is needed for a certain ingredient like HMB (beta-hydroxy-beta-methylbutyrate) that has a short half-life in the body, then a tablet is usually used because a softgel or capsule is impractical for this type of delivery. They can also have a wax coating for easy swallowing.

Softgels

Softgels are lipid-containing liquid caps that are readily absorbed. The amounts of the active ingredients can be well-controlled based on the amount found in each softgel. Liquids found within softgels can be microencapsulated for even better delivery. Most softgels contain fat-soluble ingredients such as vitamin E.

Liquids

Liquids are one of the fastest-absorbing delivery systems because they require minimal digestion. They can enter the bloodstream quickly, plus larger gram amounts of nutrients can be delivered easier. For example, when doctors perform a glucose tolerance test, they have you drink a sugary, high–glycemic index carbohydrate drink (glucose mixed with water) to elicit the maximum blood sugar response, and hence insulin response, fast. Liquids are great to take during workouts due to their quick absorption, which helps you avoid stomachaches. Liquids are also becoming popular vehicles for delivery of herbs and other dietary supplements. The "medicine-like" taste of liquid supplements is always an issue, but manufacturers are using advanced techniques like microencapsulation and liposomes to mask the taste of bitter herbs and other supplements that have an unpleasant taste. After all, if you can't stand the taste, it is highly unlikely you will take it regularly.

Liposomal Delivery System

Liposomes are microscopic spherical vesicles that form when phospholipids are hydrated. These vesicles can contain both fat- and water-soluble nutrients, which is an added bonus. Liposomal-based delivery systems have been used successfully for years by the pharmaceutical industry and have recently been showing up in nutritional supplements. They come in liquid and powdered form and can help mask the bitter taste of certain nutrients. Liposomes can be custom designed for almost any need by varying the lipid content, size, surface charge, and method of preparation. They are very stable and can deliver nutrients in a varying controlled, sustained, or timed-release manner, depending on the number of layers they contain. Liposomes can also protect oral delivery of sensitive nutrients. A few studies show a threefold increase in absorption of nutrients into the bloodstream using liposomal delivery.

Effervescent Delivery

Effervescent delivery is yet another effective way to get nutrients into the bloodstream fast (from the small intestine). Effervescent technology usually uses sodium bicarbonate and other ingredients to help buffer stomach acid and increase absorption of nutrients. This is an excellent delivery system if stomach discomfort is a concern as it seems to lower stomach problems associated with many nutrients. Nutrients that come in an effervescent delivery system include glutamine, creatine, and vitamin C.

Sublingual and Buccal Delivery

Sublingual (under the tongue) and buccal (by the mouth) delivery are also used for ingredients that need to be taken directly into the bloodstream, bypassing the digestive tract and liver completely. You see, some nutrients are not only destroyed by the harsh stomach acids and enzymes, but they are also broken down by liver enzymes as they go through the "first pass" in the liver. This may mean that only a very small amount of the ingested nutrient reaches the bloodstream and hence the target tissues like the muscles. Bypassing this process can allow for sensitive nutrients to get into the bloodstream fast. This is usually a liquid delivery that has to be taken under the tongue for absorption into the oral cavity and then the lymphatic system, which allows nutrients to be absorbed more quickly into the bloodstream.

Be aware that some nutrients that are taken orally simply cannot be taken sublingually due to their molecular size. This is a rather limited delivery system, but one advantage is that since there is a very high absorption rate of nutrients directly into the bloodstream, a smaller amount of certain nutrients can be used. This may help make some nutrients more cost-effective.

Other Forms

Other delivery systems, such as enteric-coated tablets (a film coating that protects sensitive nutrients from the harsh environment of the stomach) and nasal absorption, are less common. Balancing the pH or buffering nutrients is also available, although the jury is still out on the science of this practice. And some of the earliest use of prohormones was through a nasal spray delivery system.

How Sports Supplements Are Created

I'm sure many sports supplement company executives will not be thrilled about this chapter. This is the part of the book that describes how sports supplements end up on the shelf at your local health food store or on the Internet. Like everything else, there is a right way and a wrong way to do things. Credible sports supplement companies generally do a lot of homework and have processes and procedures in place to develop new products. These quality companies don't throw out supplements left and right just to copy a hot-selling item—no, they actually try to create cutting-edge products so that you, the supplement consumer, can reach your goals of getting bigger, leaner, stronger, and more energetic.

The Bad and the Ugly

These days, the "me too" products are a dime a dozen. Anytime there is a hot-selling supplement, ten companies will quickly launch similar products using lower quality ingredients to make the price cheaper. One example of this is the NO (nitric oxide)-boosting products containing the amino acid L-arginine. Everyone jumped on that bandwagon. Copying products is bad enough, but when companies cut costs by using cheap, low-grade ingredients, the consumer loses out. Copying products doesn't take much skill, and since there is no pre-approval of products (although there is for new individual dietary ingredients) by the U.S. Food and Drug Administration (FDA), anybody with a little knowledge of the industry and a few bucks can quickly launch a similar product on the market.

One inside secret is that some companies are actually approached by retail chains to develop certain types of products. The reason that these retail chains approach a company to develop a certain line of products is because they are having a disagreement or a falling out with a brand they carry and they now want to replace it. For example, let's say retail chain A carries BigMuscle products but they have a disagreement. Well, retail chain A will approach company B to develop the same products as BigMuscle and then use this against BigMuscle to negotiate a better deal. This will either drive out BigMuscle products from their store or cause BigMuscle to meet the demands of retail chain A—which usually means selling to them for a cheaper price. It's always about the money. . . .

The Good

Okay, enough of the negativity—there are many companies who develop and market products the right way, the way that instills confidence in consumers like you. The following is a step-by-step guide on how quality products are created.

1. Ideation—In this initial phase of the product development process, a lot of brainstorming takes place and supplement concepts are passed by company employees and focus groups. A need will be established—such as boosting testosterone levels, for example—and then a product will be thought out to address that need. This step allows the developers to establish the desired claims for a product—what they will say about the product and the claims they will make. This phase also determines who the product is targeted toward and how to reach that group in an effective manner. Experts will be utilized during this step to get feedback and ideas, and some of these experts may even become endorsers of the product.

2. Formula—After coming up with a product concept, a theoretical formula is generally submitted to the Research and Development (R&D) group with targeted claims. This includes the exact ingredients in the product. Published clinical research supporting each ingredient in the product is also collected.

3. Packaging—Various types of packaging are looked at and reviewed. The amount of product per bottle will also be determined at this time. For example, 120 tablets for a one month supply. Graphics people start coming up with a label design and put some branding concepts into it.

4. Marketing Information—Information describing the product in detail will be created, including advertisements, sales sheets, research information, and other material that supports selling the product. Some teaser ads will go out in print and on the Internet. This helps test the products to see if they will sell. Graphics people spruce all this up to increase marketability. This is the stage where credible, legitimate companies who use trustworthy scientific-based claims in their marketing are separated from those companies who are not so credible. The not-so-credible companies may highly exaggerate their product claims in order to get you to buy their products, over others, even if that means telling outright lies.

5. Formulation Development—All the raw materials will be sourced out and the formula is sent to their preferred manufacturers (unless the company manufactures its own products) to determine costs. The final cost of the formula is determined and the appropriate cost at the wholesale and retail level will be established for the supplement. A preliminary stability test will also be performed at this stage.

6. Testing—Sample batches of the product are made and tested on a sampling of people. Results from these tests are gathered and reviewed. Research centers are contacted to do a more thorough clinical study on the product itself and a pilot study usually will be initiated.

7. Production Scale-Up—Another sample batch will be made up so that it can be tested in the laboratory to make sure it meets the label claims and to ensure that the product is stable over the long term. An expiration date is also determined, generally two to three years from the manufacturing date as long as the product is stored in a cool, dry place.

8. Regulatory—The label claims and all the marketing materials are submitted to an FDA and Federal Trade Commission (FTC) specialist (usually an attorney) for approval. If some of the claims are unsubstantiated, then the marketing material has to be re-worked and the label revised. Some attorneys allow more claims than others. This step includes adding the product to the company's insurance policy.

9. Final Approval of the Formula—Once the pilot batch and the marketing claims are approved and the study validates their claims for safety and effectiveness, the product will be signed off on by the appropriate management personnel.

10. Production and Shipment—The R&D team will generally monitor the production of the first batch of product. Then, the product is shipped and appears on the retail shelf or on the Internet.

That is how a high-quality product is produced. This process takes extra time and money, but credible companies feel it is well worth it in the long run. Beginning on page 206 is a list of the quality, reputable companies we recommend.

How to Buy
Sports Supplements

Read the Supplement Facts Label

When buying supplements, it is important to look at the "Supplement Facts" label (for meal replacement or protein powders, it is usually called "Nutrition Facts"). Important things to look for include the following:

1. Reasonable serving size—Make sure the product contains a serving size that allows you to get at least a 20–30 day supply per bottle. This should be listed as "servings per container." Some unscrupulous supplement companies promise a month's supply per bottle, but when you examine the label closely you find it only contains a 10–15 day supply based on the recommended dosage. Watch out for this "serving size" game.

2. Patent numbers and branded ingredient logos—If ingredients in a product are branded, such as 7-Keto® and Forslean®, it usually means that more research has been done on them. Although patent numbers listed on the bottle don't guarantee the effectiveness of the product, it is usually a sign that the company spent a lot of time, energy, and "extra" money in developing the product and it has something unique.

3. Standardized herbs—If the product contains herbs, make sure they are standardized to their active ingredient (the word *standardized* should appear). For example, green tea should be standardized for at least 40 percent EGCG (epigallocatechin gallate) for fat loss. This standardization insures the full potency of the herb.

4. Research references—Although this is not commonplace, some quality products have published research study references (not pilot studies) list-

ed on the label. An example of what this might look like is: Aagaard, P., et al. *Med Sci Sports Exerc* 38:5 Suppl (2006): S9.

5. Company contact information—The label should list the address, phone number, and website of the company.

Finding Reputable Supplement Companies

With so many sports supplements and supplement manufacturers out there, it is important to understand what to look for in a quality company, especially in this industry of wheelers and dealers who just want to make a quick buck. Here is what we suggest you look for:

Excellent quality control. This means the company uses either an U.S. Food and Drug Administration (FDA)–licensed or cGMP (current good manufacturing practices)–approved manufacturer. They should be able to give you this information over the phone or via e-mail. They should also have current laboratory analyses of their products confirming the purity of their ingredients (make sure they don't send you outdated information). Reputable companies use high-quality raw material suppliers that test for impurities in their ingredients, especially herbs.

Real research. There are only a handful of companies that fund independent clinical research studies on their specific products. This is a good sign that the company is legitimate, because this process can be a costly endeavor. Quality companies allow this research to be published or presented at a scientific conference no matter what the outcome, good *or* bad. They should be willing to provide you with a copy of the actual study, the abstract, or the pubmed link. Companies looking to cut corners will "borrow" another company's research and claim it to be their own. They might also choose to hide or not publish funded research that doesn't show the results they were hoping to achieve. Be very cautious of "in-house" research or pilot studies that are not even being considered for peer-reviewed publication. Also, it's a good idea to be skeptical of most testimonials unless you've seen the results with your own eyes in a friend or family member.

Information provider. A solid company also provides quality nutrition and training information via their website and/or information booklets. They give the user of their products more than just a pill or powder—rather, it's a complete plan for success.

Real money-back guarantee. Although many companies have a guarantee of some sort, look for an unconditional money-back guarantee that is honored by the company. In other words, if you use their product over a specific period of time and don't get the results you were promised, then they should have no problem giving you a full refund without a hassle. Quality companies realize that this is a small minority and want to give the consumer their money back if the product doesn't work. Watch out for "limited" money-back guarantees or statements such as "all sales are final." Read the fine print and ask questions—it's your hard-earned money at stake.

Freedom of information. The company should have nothing to hide and can provide any of the above items without a problem. A simple phone call or e-mail to the company should allow you to get all your questions answered. If the company doesn't list the amount of an ingredient on the label, they should be able to tell you the amount (or at least a good range) of that specific ingredient over the phone or through e-mail. If they can't, that might tell you something about their credibility.

Fairly credible advertisements. Most reputable companies tell the truth in their marketing materials, promise attainable results using their products, and provide a solid nutrition and training program. Of course, there is nothing wrong with clever marketing (companies have to make money, after all). "Gain 20 pounds of muscle in two weeks"—just remember, if it sounds too good to be true, it probably is.

Well thought-out products. Reputable companies produce products with some good reasoning behind them. Don't trust "kitchen sink" formulas that can do everything for you. Look for targeted formulas with a credible explanation for the inclusion of each ingredient.

Of course, there are other factors besides these in determining if a company has reputable products. In fact, it can even vary from product to product (that is, some companies have a great protein powder but a lower-quality fat burner). For those of us who have been involved in the industry for the past 15 years, there is also something to say about the credibility of people who are running the company—credible people usually run credible companies.

Some Top Sports Supplement Companies

BSN

One of the true success stories in the sports nutrition industry, BSN is headed by people who know about training and the supplement industry. They have good products and provide easy-to-use programs on their website. They also shook up the industry by signing some of the most sought after athletes, including Mr. Olympia Ronnie Coleman and fitness expert Monica Brant. Their products include Nitrix, NO Xplode, and Syntha-6.

Tel: 877-431-9574 • Website: www.bsnonline.net

EAS (Experimental and Applied Sciences)

EAS is one of the true leaders and pioneers in the supplement industry. It is now owned by Abbott Laboratories and focuses on athletes and sports leagues, including the NFL. The company provides useful products and meets most if not all of the above criteria. EAS has funded a lot of clinical research and provided numerous educational programs. They have excellent products for people from all walks of life. EAS makes one of the top meal replacement products (Myoplex Original and Myoplex Deluxe) and cutting-edge products like Muscle Armor and C3. The product quality is very high and the credibility of this company is solid.

555 Corporate Circle
Golden, CO 80401
Tel: 800-297-9776 • Fax: 303-279-6465 • Website: www.eas.com

iSatori Technologies

This customer-friendly company is run by co-author, Stephen Adelé, an avid weight trainer and supplement industry expert. iSatori is one of the very few companies that conducts independent clinical studies on all of their products. They also provide consumers with free, customized diet and weight-training plans (in published books and downloads on their website) to help them achieve their fitness goals. Adelé also runs *Real Solutions* magazine, which provides practical, up-to-date information on nutrition, training, and supplementation by some of the leading experts in the field. iSatori products include Lean System 7, 3-XL, Isa-Test, Eat-Smart, Energize, MX-LS7, and H-Blocker.

15000 W. 6th Avenue, Suite 202
Golden, CO 80401
Tel: 866-688-7679 • Fax: 303-215-1386 • Website: www.isatoritech.com

Labrada

Bodybuilding legend Lee Labrada owns this company, which has proven to be very ethical and trustworthy. Their products include Lean Body bars and meal replacement products. Labrada is also great about consumer education, with an online coaching club to help people get the body of their dreams.

Tel: 800-832-9948 • Website: www.labrada.com

MHP (Maximum Human Performance)

MHP is run by a former top bodybuilder named Gerard Dente. The company utilizes doctors and other experts in their development of science-based products. Their products including T-Bomb II, Anadrox, and TRAC Extreme NO.

1376 Pompton Avenue
Cedar Grove, NJ 07009
Tel: 888-783-8844 • Website: www.maxperformance.com

Muscle-Link

This is a reputable company with solid, targeted products and associated with *Ironman* magazine. It is run by some of the most honest people in the supplement industry. Some of their products are Muscle Meals (an MRP), Pro-Fusion, Cort-Bloc, and Recover-X (a post-workout recovery drink).

1701 Ives Avenue
Oxnard, CA 93033
Tel: 800-570-4766

MuscleTech

MuscleTech Research and Development is a company based in Canada that has targeted sports nutrition products for the bodybuilder and fitness enthusiast alike. They are sometimes criticized for their "hyped-up" marketing claims, but they have good products that are based on solid scientific research. They have clinical studies from credible research facilities, laboratory analysis of all their products confirming the purity of the ingredients, and a user-friendly website. Their products include Nitro-Tech, Hydroxycut, and Cell-Tech, plus a host of cutting-edge products like Leukic and naNO^{X9}.

Iovate Health Sciences U.S.A. Inc.
3880 Jeffrey Blvd.
Blasdell, NY 14219
Tel: 877-443-4074 • Website: www.muscletech.com

NX Labs

This Canadian company is one of the new kids on the block (with many former employees of MuscleTech working in the company). Their products are very cutting-edge and potent. They also provide lots of information in terms of training and diet with books and websites for some of their individual products.

Tel: 877-695-2271 • Website: www.nxlabs.com

SAN

This company has innovative products that keep pushing the envelope. It is run by Matt Boldt, who is very knowledgeable about the science of supplements. Some of their solid products include Tight, Fierce, and Triple Strength Fish Fats.

716 N. Ventura Road #431
Oxnard, CA 93030
Tel: 888-519-9300 • Website: www.sann.net

References

The Importance of Whole Foods

Borkman, M., et al. "The Relationship Between Insulin Sensitivity and the Fatty Acid Composition of Skeletal-muscle Phospholipids." *N Engl J Med* 328 (1993): 238–244.

Dorgan, J., et al. "Effects of Dietary Fat and Fiber on Plasma and Urine Androgens and Estrogens in Men: A Controlled Feeding Study." *Am J Clin Nutr* 64:6 (1996): 850–855.

Dray, F., et al. "Role of Prostaglandins on Growth Hormone Secretion: PGE2, a Physiological Stimulator." *Adv Prostaglandin Thromboxane Res* 8 (1980): 1321–1328.

Erasmus, Udo. *Fats That Heal, Fats That Kill.* Burnaby, BC, Canada: Alive Books, 1993.

Garg, M., et al. "Fish Oil Prevents Change in Arachidonic Acid and Cholesterol Content in Rat Caused by Dietary Cholesterol." *Lipids* 24:4 (1989): 266–270.

Groff, J., S. Gropper, and S. Hunt. *Advanced Nutrition and Human Metabolism,* 2nd ed. St. Paul, MN: West, 1995.

Guarner, F. "Inulin and Oligofructose: Impact on Intestinal Diseases and Disorders." *Br J Nutr* 93:Suppl 1 (2005): S61–S65.

Hamalainen, E., et al. "Diet and Serum Sex Hormones in Healthy Men." *J Steroid Biochem* 20:1 (1984): 459–464.

Lemon, Peter. "Is Increased Dietary Protein Necessary or Beneficial for Individuals with a Physically Active Lifestyle." *Nutr Rev* 54 (1996): S169–S175.

Liang, T., and S. Liao. "Inhibition of Steroid 5 Alpha-reductase by Specific Aliphatic Unsaturated Fatty Acids." *J Biochem* 285:Part 2 (1992): 557–562.

Marlett, J.A., et al. "The Active Fraction of Psyllium Seed Husk." *Proc Nutr Soc* 62:1 (2003): 207–209.

Sebokova, E., et al. "Alteration of the Lipid Composition of Rat Testicular Plasma Membranes by Dietary (n-3) Fatty Acids Changes the Responsiveness of Leydig Cells and Testosterone Synthesis." *J Nutr* 120:6 (1990): 610–618.

Tipton, K., et al. "Exercise, Protein Metabolism, and Muscle Growth." *Int J Sport Nutr Exerc Metab* 11:1 (2001): 109–132.

Tokunaga, K., and A. Matsuoka. "Effects of a [FOSHU] Which Contains Indigestible Dextrin as an Effective Ingredient on Glucose and Lipid Metabolism." *J Japan Diabetes Soc* 42 (1999): 61–65.

Volek, J., W. Kraemer, J. Bush, et al. "Testosterone and Cortisol in Relationship to Dietary Nutrients and Resistance Exercise." *J Appl Physiol* 82:1 (1997): 49–54.

Warner, J., et al. "Combined Effects of Aerobic Exercise and Omega-3 Fatty-acids on Plasma Lipids in Hyperlipidemic Subjects." *Clin Res* 34:2 (1986): 806A.

Protein Powders and Nutrition Bars

Allison, D.B., et al. "A Novel Soy-based Meal Replacement Formula for Weight Loss Among Obese Individuals: A Randomized Controlled Clinical Trial." *Eur J Clin Nutr* 57:4 (2003): 514–522.

Arnold, L.M., et al. "Effect of Isoenergetic Intake of Three or Nine Meals on Plasma Lipoproteins and Glucose Metabolism." *Am J Clin Nutr* 57:3 (1993): 446–451.

Boire, Y., et al. "Slow and Fast Dietary Proteins Differently Modulate Postprandial Protein Accretion." *Proc Natl Acad Sci USA* 94:26 (1997): 14930–14935.

Brown, E.C., et al. "Soy versus Whey Protein Bars: Effects on Exercise Training Impact on Lean Body Mass and Antioxidant Status." *Nutr J* 3:1 (2004): 22.

Demling, R.H., et al. "Effect of a Hypocaloric Diet, Increased Protein Intake and Resistance Training on Lean Mass Gains and Fat Mass Loss in Overweight Police Officers." *Ann Nutr Metab* 44:1 (2000): 21–29.

Desroches, S., et al. "Effects of Dietary Conjugated Linoleic Acid on Plasma Lipoproteins and Body Composition in Obese Men." *Obesity Res* 9 Suppl 3 (2001): 87S–87S.

Doi, T., T. Matsuo, M. Sugawara, et al. "New Approach for Weight Reduction by a Combination of Diet, Light Resistance Exercise and the Timing of Ingesting a Protein Supplement." *Asia Pacific J Clin Nutr* 10:3 (2001): 226–232.

Kalman, D., et al. "A Randomized Double-Blind Clinical Pilot Trial Evaluating the Effect of Protein Source when Combined with Resistance Training on Body Composition and Sex Hormones in Adult Males." Presented at the Experimental Biology Conference 2005, San Diego, California.

Khalil, D., et al. "Soy Protein Supplementation Increases Serum Insulin-like Growth Factor-1 in Young and Old Men but Does Not Affect Markers of Bone Metabolism." *J Nutr* 132:9 (2002): 2605–2608.

Le Blanc. J., et al. "Components of Postprandial Thermogenesis in Relation to Meal Frequency in Humans." *Can J Physiol Pharmacol* 71:12 (1993): 879–883.

Li, Z., et al. "Long-term Efficacy of Soy-based Meal Replacements vs. an Individualized Diet Plan in Obese Type II DM Patients: Relative Effects on Weight Loss, Metabolic Parameters, and C-reactive Protein." *Eur J Clin Nutr* (December 22, 2004).

Micke, P., et al. "Oral Supplementation with Whey Proteins Increases Plasma Glutathione Levels of HIV-infected Patients." *Eur J Clin Invest* 31:2 (2001): 171–178.

Vitamins and Minerals

Alaswad, K., J.H. O'Keefe Jr., and R.M. Moe. "Combination Drug Therapy for Dyslipidemia." *Curr Atheroscler Rep* 1:1 (1999): 44–49.

Aprahamian, M., A. Dentinger, C. Stock-Damge, et al. "Effects of Supplemental Pantothenic Acid on Wound Healing: Experimental Study in Rabbit." *Am J Clin Nutr* 41:3 (1985): 578–589.

Bender, D.A. *Nutritional Biochemistry of the Vitamins.* New York: Cambridge University Press, 1992, pp. 184–222.

Bhathena, S.J., L. Recant, N.R. Voyles, et al. "Decreased Plasma Enkephalins in Copper Deficiency in Man." *Am J Clin Nutr* 43:1 (1986): 42–46.

Brilla, L.R., and T.F. Haley. "Effect of Magnesium Supplementation on Strength Training in Humans." *J Amer Coll Nutr* 11:3 (1992): 326–329.

Cook, J.D., and E.R. Monson. "Vitamin C, The Common Cold, and Iron Absorption." *Am J Clin Nutr* 30 (1977): 235–241.

Cordova, A., and M. Alvarez-Mon. "Behavior of Zinc in Physical Exercise: A Special Reference to Immunity and Fatigue." *Neurosci Biobehav Rev* 19:3 (1995): 439–445.

Englisch, R., et al. "Induction of Glucose Transport into Rat Muscle by Selenate and Selenite: Comparison to Insulin," *Diabetologia* 38:1 Suppl (1995): A133.

Groff, J., S. Gropper, and S. Hunt. *Advanced Nutrition and Human Metabolism,* 2nd ed. St. Paul, MN: West, 1995.

Heyliger, C.E., A.G. Tahiliani, and J.H. McNeill. "Effect of Vanadate on Elevated Blood Glucose and Depressed Cardiac Performance of Diabetic Rats." *Science* 227 (1985): 1474–1477.

Johnston, C.S., and B. Luo. "Comparison of the Absorption and Excretion of Three Commercially Available Sources of Vitamin C." *J Am Diet Assoc* 94 (1994): 779–781.

Katts, G., et al. "The Effects of Chromium Picolinate Supplementation on Body Composition in Different Age Groups." *Age* 14:40 (1991): 138.

Kiremidjian-Schumacher, L., and G. Stotzky. "Selenium and Immune Responses." *Environmental Res* 42:2 (1987): 277–303.

Klesges, R.C., K.D. Ward, M.L. Shelton, et al. "Changes in Bone Mineral Content in Male Athletes: Mechanisms of Action and Intervention Effects." *JAMA* 276:3 (1996): 226–230.

Lemann, J., J.A. Pless, and R.W. Gary. "Potassium Causes Calcium Retention in Healthy Adults." *J Nutr* 123 (1993): 1623–1626.

Liakakos, D., N.L. Doulas, D. Ikkos, et al. "Inhibitory Effect of Ascorbic Acid (Vitamin C) on Cortisol Secretion Following Adrenal Stimulation in Children." *Clin Chem Acta* 65:3 (1975): 251–255.

Meador, K.J. "Evidence for a Central Cholinergic Effect of High-dose Thiamine." *Ann Neurol* 34 (1993): 724–726.

Peters, E.M., R. Anderson, D.C. Nieman, et al. "Vitamin C Supplementation Attenuates the Increases in Circulating Cortisol, Adrenaline and Anti-inflammatory Polypeptides Following Ultramarathon Running." *Int J Sports Med* 22:7 (2001): 537–543.

Phillips, C.L., S.B. Combs, and S.R. Pinnell. "Effects of Ascorbic Acid on Proliferation and Collagen Synthesis in Relation to the Donor Age of Human Dermal Fibroblasts." *J Invest Dermatol* 103:2 (1994): 228–232.

Prasad, A.S., C.S. Mantzoros, F.W. Beck, et al. "Zinc Status and Serum Testosterone Levels of Healthy Adults." *Nutrition* 12:5 (1996): 344–348.

Rupp, J.C., et al. "Effect of Sodium Bicarbonate Ingestion on Blood and Muscle pH and Exercise Performance." *Med Sci Sports Exerc* 15 (1983): 115.

Suttie, J.W. "Vitamin K and Human Nutrition." *J Am Diet Assoc* 92 (1992): 585–590.

Wilkes, D., N. Gledhill, and R. Smyth. "Effect of Induced Metabolic Alkalosis on 800-m Racing Time." *Med Sci Sports Exerc* 15:4 (1983): 277–280.

Wolf, G. "Multiple Functions of Vitamin A." *Physiol Rev* 64 (1984): 873–937.

Zemel, M.B. "Role of Dietary Calcium and Dairy Products in Modulating Adiposity." *Lipids* 38:2 (2003): 139–146.

Antioxidants and Free Radicals

Alessio, H.M., et al. "Exercise-induced Oxidative Stress Before and After Vitamin C Supplementation." *Int J Sport Nutr* 7:1 (1997): 1–9.

Anderson, J.W., et al. "Selective Effects of Different Antioxidants on Oxidation of Lipoproteins from Rats." *Proc Soc Exp Biol Med* 218:4 (1998): 376–381.

Bagchi, D., et al. "Free Radicals and Grape Seed Proanthocyanidin Extract: Importance in Human Health and Disease Prevention." *Toxicology* 148:2–3 (2000): 187–197.

Benzie, I.F., et al. "Consumption of Green Tea Causes Rapid Increase in Plasma Antioxidant Power in Humans." *Nutr Cancer* 34:1 (1999): 83–87.

Cordova, A., and M. Alvarez-Mon. "Behavior of Zinc in Physical Exercise: a Special Reference to Immunity and Fatigue." *Neurosci Biobehav Rev* 19:3 (1995): 439–445.

Dardenne, M. "Zinc and Immune Function." *Eur J Clin Nutr* 56:Suppl 3 (2002): S20–S23.

Diplock, A.T. "Vitamin E." In Diplock, A.T. (ed.). *Fat-Soluble Vitamins.* Lancaster, PA: Technomic, 1984, pp. 154–224.

Gheldof, N., et al. "Antioxidant Capacity of Honeys from Various Floral Sources Based on the Determination of Oxygen Radical Absorbance Capacity and Inhibition of in vitro Lipoprotein Oxidation in Human Serum Samples." *J Agric Food Chem* 50 (2002): 3050–3055.

Hahn, F., and J. Ciak. "Berberine." *Antibiotics* 3 (1976): 577–588.

Huang, D., et al. "High-throughput Assay of Oxygen Radical Absorbance Capacity (ORAC) Using a Multichannel Liquid Handling System Coupled with a Microplate Fluorescence Reader in 96-well Format." *J Agric Food Chem* 50 (2002): 4437–4444.

Jain, A., et al. "Effect of Ascorbate or N-acetylcysteine Treatment in a Patient with Hereditary Glutathione Synthestase Deficiency." *J Pediatr* 124 (1994): 229–233.

Karlsson, J. *Antioxidants and Exercise.* Champaign, IL.: Human Kinetics, 1997.

King, J.C., and C.L. Keen. "Zinc." In Shils, M.E., J.A. Olson, and M. Shike (eds.). *Modern Nutrition in Health and Disease,* 8th ed. Philadelphia: Lea and Febiger, 1994, pp. 214–230.

Kinscherf, R., et al. "Low Plasma Glutamine in Combination with High Glutamate Levels Indicate Risk for Loss of Body Cell Mass in Healthy Individuals: The Effect of N-acetyl-cysteine." *J Mol Med* 74:7 (1996): 393–400.

Melchart, D., et al. "Echinacea Root Extracts for the Prevention of Upper Respiratory Tract Infections: A Double-Blind, Placebo-Controlled Randomized Trial." *Arch Fam Med* 7:6 (1998): 541–545.

Peters, E.M., et al. "Vitamin C Supplementation Attenuates the Increases in Circulating Cortisol, Adrenaline and Anti-inflammatory Polypeptides Following Ultra Marathon Running." *Int J Sports Med* 22:7 (2001): 537–543.

Peters, E.M., et al. "Attenuation of Increase in Circulating Cortisol and Enhancement of the Acute Phase Protein Response in Vitamin C–Supplemented Ultramarathoners." *Int J Sports Med* 22:2 (2001): 120–126.

Schroder, H., et al. "Effects of Alpha-tocopherol, Beta-carotene and Ascorbic Acid on Oxidative, Hormonal and Enzymatic Exercise Stress Markers in Habitual Training Activity of Professional Basketball Players." *Eur J Nutr* 40:4 (2001): 178–184.

Schroder, H., et al. "Nutrition Antioxidant Status and Oxidative Stress in Professional Basketball Players: Effects of a Three-compound Antioxidative Supplement." *Int J Sports Med* 21:2 (2000): 146–150.

Sjodin, B., et. al. "Biochemical Mechanisms for Oxygen Free Radical Formation During Exercise." *Sports Med* 10:4 (1990): 236–254.

Vasankari, T., et al. "Effects of Ascorbic Acid and Carbohydrate Ingestion on Exercise-induced Oxidative Stress." *J Sports Med Phys Fitness* 38 (1998): 281–285.

Essential Fatty Acids—Good Fats Can Build a Better Body

Borkman, M., et al. "The Relationship Between Insulin Sensitivity and the Fatty Acid Composition of Skeletal-muscle Phospholipids." *N Engl J Med* 328 (1993): 238–244.

Dorgan, J., et al. "Effects of Dietary Fat and Fiber on Plasma and Urine Androgens and Estrogens in Men: A Controlled Feeding Study." *Am J Clin Nutr* 64:6 (1996): 850–855.

Dray, F., et al. "Role of Prostaglandins on Growth Hormone Secretion: PGE2 a Physiological Stimulator." *Adv Prostaglandin Thromboxane Res* 8 (1980): 1321–1328.

Erasmus, U. *Fats That Heal, Fats That Kill.* Burnaby, BC, Canada: Alive Books, 1993.

Garg, M., et al. "Fish Oil Prevents Change in Arachidonic Acid and Cholesterol Content in Rat Caused by Dietary Cholesterol." *Lipids* 24:4 (1989): 266–270.

Hamalainen, E., et al. "Diet and Serum Sex Hormones in Healthy Men." *J Steroid Biochem* 20:1 (1984): 459–464.

Liang, T., and S. Liao. "Inhibition of Steroid 5-Alpha-reductase by Specific Aliphatic Unsaturated Fatty Acids." *J Biochem* 285:Part 2 (1992): 557–562.

Sebokova, E., et al. "Alteration of the Lipid Composition of Rat Testicular Plasma Membranes by Dietary (n-3) Fatty Acids Changes the Responsiveness of Leydig Cells and Testosterone Synthesis." *J Nutr* 120:6 (1990): 610–618.

Volek, J., W. Kraemer, J. Bush, et al. "Testosterone and Cortisol in Relationship to Dietary Nutrients and Resistance Exercise." *J Appl Physiol* 82:1 (1997): 49–54.

Warner, J., et al. "Combined Effects of Aerobic Exercise and Omega-3 Fatty Acids on Plasma Lipids in Hyperlipidemic Subjects." *Clin Res* 34:2 (1986): 806A.

Amino Acids—The Forgotten Weapon

Deijen, J.B., et al. "Tyrosine Improves Cognitive Performance and Reduces Blood Pressure in Cadets After One Week of a Combat Training Course." *Brain Res Bull* 48:2 (1999): 203–209.

Di Luigi, L., L. Guidetti, F. Pigozzi, et al. "Acute Amino Acids Supplementation

Enhances Pituitary Responsiveness in Athletes." *Med Sci Sports Exerc* 31:12 (1999): 1748–1754.

Griffiths, R.D. "Glutamine: Establishing Clinical Indications." *Curr Opin Clin Nutr Metab Care* 2:2 (1999): 177–182.

Hurson, M., et al. "Metabolic Effects of Arginine in a Healthy Elderly Population." *J Parenter Enteral Nutr* 19:3 (1995): 227–230.

Liu, Z., L.A. Jahn, W. Long, et al. "Branched Chain Amino Acids Activate Messenger Ribonucleic Acid Translation Regulatory Proteins in Human Skeletal Muscle, and Glucocorticoids Blunt This Action." *J Clin Endocrinol Metab* 86:5 (2001): 2136–2143.

Maclean, D.A., T.E. Graham, and B. Saltin. "Branched-chain Amino Acids Augment Ammonia Metabolism While Attenuating Protein Breakdown During Exercise." *Am J Physiol* 267:6 Part 1 (1994): E1010–E1022.

Mourier, A., A.X. Bigard, E. de Kerviler, et al. "Combined Effects of Caloric Restriction and Branched-chain Amino Acid Supplementation on Body Composition and Exercise Performance in Elite Wrestlers." *Int J Sports Med* 18:1 (1997): 47–55.

Neri, D.F., D. Wiegmann, R.R. Stanny, et al. "The Effects of Tyrosine on Cognitive Performance During Extended Wakefulness." *Aviat Space Environ Med* 66:4 (1995): 313–319.

Owasoyo, J.O., et al. "Tyrosine and Its Potential Use as a Countermeasure to Performance Decrement in Military Sustained Operations." *Aviat Space Environ Med* 63:5 (1992): 364–369.

Salter, C.A. "Dietary Tyrosine as an Aid to Stress Resistance Among Troops." *Mil Med* 154:3 (1989): 144–146.

Schaefer, A., et al. "L-arginine Reduces Exercise-induced Increase in Plasma Lactate and Ammonia." *Int J Sports Med* 23:6 (2002): 403–407.

Stein, T.P., et al. "Attenuation of the Protein Wasting Associated with Bed Rest by Branched-chain Amino Acids." *Nutrition* 15:9 (1999): 656–660.

Van Hall, G., W.H. Saris, P.A. van de Schoor, and A.J. Wagenmakers. "The Effect of Free Glutamine and Peptide Ingestion on the Rate of Muscle Glycogen Resynthesis in Man." *Int J Sports Med* 21:1 (2000): 25–30.

Welbourne, T.C. "Increased Plasma Bicarbonate and Growth Hormone After an Oral Glutamine Load." *Am J Clin Nutr* 61:5 (1995): 1058–1061.

Wolfe, R.R. "Effects of Amino Acid Intake on Anabolic Processes." *Can J Appl Physiol* 26:Suppl (2001): S220–S227.

Yaspelkis, B.B. 3rd, and J.L. Ivy. "The Effect of a Carbohydrate-Arginine Supplement on Postexercise Carbohydrate Metabolism." *Int J Sport Nutr* 9:3 (1999): 241–250.

Fat Loss: Thermogenic Supplements

Bruce, C., M. Anderson, et al. "Enhancement of 2000-m Rowing Performance After Caffeine Ingestion." *Med Sci Sports Exerc* 32:11 (2000): 1958–1963.

Colker, C., et al., "Effects of *Citrus Aurantium* Extract, Caffeine, and St. John's Wort on Body Fat Loss, Lipid Levels, and Mood States in Overweight Healthy Adults." *Curr Ther Res* 60:3 (1999): 145–153.

Doherty, M. "The Effects of Caffeine on the Maximum Accumulated Oxygen Deficit and Short-term Running Performance." *Int J Sport Nutr* 8:2 (1998): 95–104.

Dulloo, A.G., et al. "Efficacy of a Green Tea Extract Rich in Catechin Polyphenols and Caffeine in Increasing 24-h Energy Expenditure and Fat Oxidation in Humans." *Am J Clin Nutr* 70:6 (1999): 1040–1050.

Dulloo, A.G., et al. "Green Tea and Thermogenesis: Interactions Between Catechin-polyphenols, Caffeine and Sympathetic Activity." *Int J Obes Relat Metab Disord* 24:2 (2000): 252–258.

Graham, T. "Caffeine and Exercise: Metabolism, Endurance, and Performance." *Sports Med* 31:11 (2001): 785–807.

McCarty, M. "Optimizing Exercise for Fat Loss." *Med Hypotheses* 44:5 (1995): 325–330.

Nehlig, A., and G. Debry. "Caffeine and Sports Activity." *Int J Sports Med* 15:5 (1994): 215–223.

Watanabe, T., et al. "Effect of Capsaicin Pre-treatment on Capsaicin-induced Catecholamine From the Adrenal Medulla in Rats." *Proc Soc Exp Biol Med* 187 (1988): 370–374.

Yoshida, T., N. Sakane, et al. "Relationship Between Basal Metabolic Rate, Thermogenic Response to Caffeine, and Body Weight Loss Following Combined Low Calorie and Exercise Treatment in Obese Women." *Int J Obes Relat Metab Disord* 18:5 (1994): 345–350.

Non-Stimulant Fat-Loss Agents

Agarwal, R.C., S.P. Singh, R.K. Saran, et al. "Clinical Trials of Gugulipid—A New Hypolipidemic Agent of Plant Origin in Primary Hyperlipidemia." *Indian J Med Res* 84 (1986): 626–634.

Belury, M.A., A. Mahon, and S. Banni. "The Conjugated Linoleic Acid (CLA) Isomer, t10c12-CLA, is Inversely Associated with Changes in Body Weight and Serum Leptin in Subjects with Type 2 Diabetes Mellitus." *J Nutr* 133:1 (2003): 257S–260S.

Desroches, S., et al. "Effects of Dietary Conjugated Linoleic Acid on Plasma Lipoproteins and Body Composition in Obese Men." *Obesity Res* 9:Suppl 3 (2001): 87S.

Gaullier, J.M., G. Berven, H. Blankson, and O. Gudmundsen. "Clinical Trial Results Support a Preference for Using CLA Preparations Enriched with Two Isomers Rather than Four Isomers in Human Studies." *Lipids* 37:11 (2003): 1019–1025.

Gopal, K., R.K. Saran, S. Nityanand, et al. "Clinical Trial of Ethyl Acetate Extract of Gum Gugulu (Gugulipid) in Primary Hyperlipidemia." *J Assoc Physicians India* 34:4 (1986): 249–251.

Gorostiaga, E.M., C.A. Maurer, and J.P. Eclache. "Decrease in Respiratory Quotient During Exercise Following L-carnitine Supplementation." *Int J Sports Med* 10:3 (1989): 169–174.

Heymsfield, S.B., D.B. Allison, J.R. Vasselli, et al. "*Garcinia cambogia* (Hydroxycitric Acid) as a Potential Antiobesity Agent: A Randomized Controlled Trial." *JAMA* 280:18 (1998): 1596–1600.

Kaciuba-Uscilko, H., K. Nazar, J. Chwalbinska-Moneta, et al. "Effect of Phosphate Supplementation on Metabolic and Neuroendocrine Responses to Exercise and Oral Glucose Load in Obese Women During Weight Reduction." *J Physiol Pharmacol* 44:4 (1993): 425–440.

Kalman, D., et al. "A Randomized, Double-Blind, Placebo Controlled Study of 3-Acetyl-7-Oxo-Dehydroepiandrosterone in Healthy Overweight Adults." *Curr Ther Res* 61:7 (2000): 435–442.

Kamphuis, M.M., M.P. Lejeune, W.H. Saris, and M.S. Westerterp-Plantenga. "The Effect of Conjugated Linoleic Acid Supplementation after Weight Loss on Body Weight Regain, Body Composition, and Resting Metabolic Rate in Overweight Subjects." *Int J Obes Relat Metab Disord* 27:7 (2003): 840–847.

Khajuria, A., U. Zutshi, and K.L. Bedi. "Permeability Characteristics of Piperine on Oral Absorption—An Active Alkaloid from Peppers and a Bioavailability Enhancer." *Indian J Exp Biol* 36:1 (1998): 46–50.

Laurenza, A., E.M. Sutkowski, and K.B. Seamon. "Forskolin: A Specific Stimulator of Adenylyl Cyclase or a Diterpene with Multiple Sites of Action?" *Trends Pharmacol Sci* 10:11 (1989): 442–447.

Lee, E.B., et al. "Pharmacological Study on Piperine." *Arch Pharmac Res* 7 (1984): 127–132.

Muller, D.M., H. Seim, W. Kiess, et al. "Effects of Oral L-carnitine Supplementation on In Vivo Long-chain Fatty Acid Oxidation in Healthy Adults." *Metabolism* 51:11 (2002): 1389–1391.

Nazar, K., H. Kaciuba-Uscilko, J. Szczepanik, et al. "Phosphate Supplementation Prevents a Decrease of Triiodothyronine and Increases Resting Metabolic Rate During Low Energy Diet." *J Physiol Pharmacol* 47:2 (1996): 373–383.

Nityanand, S., J.S. Srivastava, and O.P. Asthana. "Clinical Trials with Gugulipid. A New Hypolipidaemic Agent." *J Assoc Physicians India* 37:5 (1989): 323–328.

Pauly, D.F., and C.J. Pepine. "The Role of Carnitine in Myocardial Dysfunction." *Am J Kidney Dis* 41:4 Suppl 4 (2003): S35–S43.

Preuss, H.G., D. Bagchi, C.V.S. Rao, et al. "Effect of Hydroxycitric Acid on Weight Loss, Body Mass Index and Plasma Leptin Levels in Human Subjects." *FASEB Journal* 16 (2002): A1020, Abstract 742.16.

Villani, R.G., J. Gannon, M. Self, and P.A. Rich. "L-Carnitine Supplementation Combined with Aerobic Training Does Not Promote Weight Loss in Moderately Obese Women." *Int J Sport Nutr Exerc Metab* 10:2 (2000): 199–207.

Volek, J.S., W.J. Kraemer, M.R. Rubin, et al. "L-Carnitine L-Tartrate Supplementation Favorably Affects Markers of Recovery From Exercise Stress." *Am J Physiol Endocrinol Metab* 282:2 (2002): E474–E482.

Wang X, et al. "The Hypolipidemic Natural Product *Commiphora mukul* and Its Component Guggulsterone Inhibit Oxidative Modification of LDL." Atherosclerosis 172:2 (2004): 239-246.

Westerterp-Plantenga, M.S., and E.M. Kovacs. "The Effects of (-)-Hydroxycitrate on Energy Intake and Satiety and in Overweight Humans." *Int J Obes Relat Metab Disord* 26:6 (2002): 870–872.

Muscle Building

Brillon, D.J., B. Zheng, R.G. Campbell, and D.E. Matthews. "Effect of Cortisol on Energy Expenditure and Amino Acid Metabolism in Humans." *Am J Physiol* 268 (1995): E501–E513.

Griffin, J., and S. Ojeda. *Textbook of Endocrine Physiology,* 3rd ed. New York: Oxford University Press, 1996.

Kelley, G.S. "*Rhodiola rosea:* A Possible Plant Adaptogen." *Altern Med Rev* 6:3 (2001): 293–302.

Simmons, P.S., J.M. Miles, J.E. Gerich, et al. "Increased Proteolysis: An Effect of Increases in Plasma Cortisol Within the Physiological Range." *J Clin Invest* 73 (1984): 412–420.

Carnosine

Amend, J.F., D.H. Strumeyer, and H. Fisher. "Effect of Dietary Histidine on Tissue Concentrations of Histidine-containing Dipeptides in Adult Cockerels." *J Nutr* 109 (1979): 1779–1786.

Bump, K.D., L.M. Lawrence, L.R. Moss, et al. "Muscle Carnosine Levels During Training and Exercise." In *Proc 11th Eq Nutr Physiol Symp* 35 (1989).

Crush, K.G. "Carnosine-related Substances in Animal Tissues." *Comp Biochem Physiol* 34 (1970): 3–30.

Dunnett, M., and R.C. Harris. "Influence of Oral Beta-Alanine and L-Histidine Supplementation on the Carnosine Content of Gluteus Medius." *Equine Vet J* 30 (1999): 499–504.

Easter, R.A., and D.H. Baker. "Nitrogen Metabolism, Tissue Carnosine Concentration and Blood Chemistry of Gravid Swine Fed Graded Levels of Histidine." *J Nutr* (1970): 120–125.

Harris, R.C., M. Dunnett, and P.L. Greenhaff. "Carnosine and Taurine contents in Individual Fibres of Human Vastus Lateralis Muscle." *J Sport Sci* 16 (1998): 639–643.

Maynard, M.L., G.A. Bossonneault, C.K. Chow, and G.A. Bruckner. "High Levels of Dietary Carnosine are Associated with Increased Concentrations of Carnosine and in Rat Soleous Muscle." *J Nutr* 131 (2001): 287–290.

Parkhouse, W.S., D.C. McKenzie, and P.W. Hochacha. "Buffering Capacity of Deproteinised Human Vastus Lateralis Muscle." *J Appl Physiol* 58 (1995): 14–17.

Suyama, M., T. Suzuki, M. Maruyama, and K. Saito. "Determination of Carnosine, Anserine and B-alanine in the Muscle of Animals." *Bull Japan Soc Sci Fish* 36 (1970): 1048–1053.

Suzuki, Y., O. Ito, N. Mukai, et al. "High Levels of Skeletal Muscle Carnosine Contributes to the Latter Half of Exercise Performance during 30s Maximal Cycle Ergometer Sprinting." *Japan J Physiol* 52:2 (2002): 199–205.

Tallon, M.J., and R.C. Harris. "Carnosine Contents in the Vastus lateralis of Extremely Hypertrophic Muscle." *Med Sci Sports Exerc* (2002).

Creatine

Almada, A., et al. "Ingestion of Creatine Serum Has No Effect on Plasma Creatine." IMAGINutrition, Inc./MetaResponses Sciences, School of Sports Studies, University College Chichester, Chichester, U.K.

Almada, A., et al. "Long-Term Creatine Supplementation Does Not Affect Markers of Renal Stress in Athletes." Presented at the 23rd National Strength and Conditioning Association Meeting, Orlando, FL, June 23, 2000.

Balsom, P.D., et al. "Creatine in Humans with Special Reference to Creatine Supplementation." *Sports Med* 18:4 (1994): 268–280.

Balsom, P.D., et al. "Skeletal Muscle Metabolism During Short Duration High-Intensity Exercise: Influence of Creatine Supplementation." *Acta Physiol Scand* 154:3 (1995): 303–310.

Birch, R., et al. "The Influence of Dietary Creatine Supplementation on Performance During Repeated Bouts of Maximal Isokinetic Cycling in Man." *Eur J Sports Nutr* 6 (1996): 222–233.

Broca, C., et al. "4-Hydroxyisoleucine: Experimental Evidence of its Insulinotropic and Antidiabetic Properties." *Am J Physiol* 277:4 Part 1 (1999): E617–E623.

Broca, C., et al. "4-Hydroxyisoleucine: Effects of Synthetic and Natural Analogues on Insulin Secretion." *Eur J Pharmacol* 390:3 (2000): 339–345.

Casey, A., et al. "Creatine Ingestion Favorably Affects Performance and Muscle Metabolism During Maximal Exercise in Humans." *Am J Physiol* 271 (1996): E31–E37.

Engelhardt, M., et al. "Creatine Supplementation in Endurance Sports." *Med Sci Sports Exerc* 30 (1998): 1123–1129.

Green, A.L., et al. "Carbohydrate Ingestion Augments Skeletal Muscle Creatine Accumulation During Creatine Supplementation in Humans." *Am J Physiol* 271:5 Part 1 (1996): E821–E826.

Greenhaff, P.L., et al. "Influence of Oral Creatine Supplementation of Torque During Repeated Bouts of Maximal Voluntary Exercise in Man." *Clin Sci* 84:5 (1993): 565–571.

Greenwood, M., et al. "Creatine Supplementation Does Not Increase Incidence of Cramping or Injury During College Football Training II." Presented at the 22nd Annual National Strength & Conditioning Association Meeting, Kansas City, MO, June 25, 1999.

Greenwood, M., et al. "D-Pinitol Augments Whole Body Creatine Retention in Man." *J Exerc Physiol Online* 4:4 (2001).

Grindstaff, P.D., et al. "Effects of Creatine Supplementation on Repetitive Sprint Performance and Body Composition in Competitive Swimmers." *Int J Sport Nutr* 7 (1997): 330–346.

Harris, R.C., et al. "Elevation of Creatine in Resting and Exercised Muscle of Normal Subjects by Creatine Supplementation." *Clin Sci* 83 (1992): 367–374.

Hespel, P., et al., "Opposite Actions of Caffeine and Creatine on Muscle Relaxation Time in Humans," J. Appl. Physiol. 92.2 (2002) : 513-518.

Juhn, M.S. "Oral Creatine Supplementation." *Physician Sports Med* 27:5 (1999).

Kelly, V.G., and D.G. Jenkins. "Effect of Oral Creatine Supplementation on Near-Maximal Strength and Repeated Sets of High-Intensity Bench Press Exercise." *J Strength Cond Res* 12 (1998): 109–115.

Kreider, R.B., et al. "Creatine Supplementation: Analysis of Ergogenic Value, Medical Safety, and Concerns." *J Exerc Physiol Online* 1:1 (1998).

Kreider, R.B., et al. "Effects of Creatine Supplementation on Body Composition, Strength and Sprint Performance." *Med Sci Sports Exerc* 30 (1998): 73–82.

Kreider, R.B. "Effects of Creatine Supplementation on Performance and Training Adaptations." Presented at the 6th International Meeting on Guanidino Compounds in Biology & Medicine, Cincinnati, OH, September 1, 2001.

Lemon, P., et al. "Effect of Oral Creatine Supplementation on Energetics During Repeated Maximal Muscle Contraction." *Med Sci Sports Exerc* 27 (1995): S204.

Passwater, R.A. *Creatine.* New Canaan, CT: Keats, 1997.

Pearson, D.R., et al. "Long-Term Effects of Creatine Monohydrate on Strength and Power." *J Strength Cond Res* 13 (1999): 187–192.

Nelson, A.G., et al. "Creatine Supplementation Raises Anaerobic Threshold." *FASEB* J 11 (1997): A589.

Sauvaire, Y., et al. "4-Hydroxyisoleucine: A Novel Amino Acid Potentiator of Insulin Secreation." *Diabetes* 47:2 (1998): 206–210

Steenge, G.R., et al. "Protein- and Carbohydrate-Induced Augmentation of Whole Body Creatine Retention in Humans." *J Appl Physiol* 89:3 (2000): 1165–1171.

Stout, J.R., et al. "The Effects of a Supplement Designed to Augment Creatine Uptake on Exercise Performance and Fat-Free Mass in Football Players." *Med Sci Sports Exerc* 29:5 (1997): S251.

Terjung, R.L., et al. "The Physiological and Health Effects of Oral Creatine Supplementation." *Med Sci Sports Exerc* 32.3 (2000): 706–717.

Vanakoski, J., et al. "Creatine and Caffeine in Anaerobic and Aerobic Exercise: Effects on Physical Performance and Pharmacokinetic Considerations." *Int J Clin Pharmacol Ther* 36:5 (1998): 258–262.

Vandenberghe, K., et al. "Caffeine Counteracts the Ergogenic Action of Muscle Creatine Loading." *J Appl Physiol* 80:2 (1996): 452–457.

Volek, J.S., et al. "Performance and Muscle Fiber Adaptations to Creatine Supplementation and Heavy Resistance Training." *Med Sci Sports Exerc* 31 (1999): 1147–1156.

Volek, J.S., et al. "Physiological Responses to Short-Term Exercise in the Heat After Creatine Loading." *Med Sci Sports Exerc* 33 (2001): 1101–1108.

Energy and Endurance

Deijen, J.B., et al. "Tyrosine Improves Cognitive Performance and Reduces Blood Pressure in Cadets After One Week of a Combat Training Course." *Brain Res Bull* 48:2 (1999): 203–209.

Dulloo, A.G., et al. "Efficacy of a Green Tea Extract Rich in Catechin Polyphenols and Caffeine in Increasing 24-h Energy Expenditure and Fat Oxidation in Humans." *Am J Clin Nutr* 70:6 (1999): 1040–1045.

Hogervost, E., W. Riedel, et al. "Caffeine Improves Cognitive Performance After Strenuous Physical Exercise." *Int J Sports Med* 20:6 (1999): 354–361.

Kelley, G.S." *Rhodiola rosea:* A Possible Plant Adaptogen." *Altern Med Rev* 6:3 (2001): 293–302.

Minehan, M.R., M.D. Riley, and L.M. Burke. "Effect of Flavor and Awareness of Kilojoule Content of Drinks on Preference and Fluid Balance in Team Sports." *Int J Sports Nutr Exerc Metabol* 12:1 (2002): 81–92.

Montner, P., D.M. Stark, M.L. Riedesel, et al. "Pre-exercise Glycerol Hydration Improves Cycling Endurance Time." *Int J Sports Med* 17:1 (1996): 27–33.

Neri, D.F., et al. "The Effects of Tyrosine on Cognitive Performance During Extended Wakefulness." *Aviat Space Environ Med* 66:4 (1995): 313–319.

Owasoyo, J.O., et al. "Tyrosine and Its Potential Use as a Countermeasure to Performance Decrement in Military Sustained Operations." *Aviat Space Environ Med* 63:5 (1992): 364–369.

Paleologos, M., et al. "Cohort Study of Vitamin C Intake and Cognitive Impairment." *Am J Epidemiol* 148:1 (1998): 45–50.

Reyner, L., and J. Horne. "Early Morning Driver Sleepiness: Effectiveness of 200 mg Caffeine." *Psychophysiology* 37:2 (2000): 251–256.

Robergs, R.A., and S.E. Griffin. "Glycerol: Biochemistry, Pharmacokinetics and Clinical and Practical Applications." *Sports Med* 26:3 (1998): 145–167.

Salter, C.A. "Dietary Tyrosine as an Aid to Stress Resistance Among Troops." *Mil Med* 154:3 (1989): 144–146.

Schroder, H., E. Navarro, J. Mora, et al. "Effects of Alpha-tocopherol, Beta-carotene and Ascorbic Acid on Oxidative, Hormonal and Enzymatic Exercise Stress Markers in Habitual Training Activity of Professional Basketball Players." *Eur J Nutr* 40:4 (2001): 178–184.

Veerendra Kumar, M.H., and Y.K. Gupta. "Effect of Different Extracts of *Centella asiatica* on Cognition and Markers of Oxidative Stress in Rats." *J Ethnopharmacol* 79:2 (2002): 253–260.

Wenos, D.L., and H.K. Amato. "Weight Cycling Alters Muscular Strength and Endurance, Ratings of Perceived Exertion, and Total Body Water in College Wrestlers." *Percept Motor Skills* 87:3 Part 1 (1998): 975–978.

Yoshida, T., et al. "Relationship Between Basal Metabolic Rate, Thermogenic Response to Caffeine, and Body Weight Loss Following Combined Low Calorie and Exercise Treatment in Obese Women." *Int J Obes Relat Metab Disord* 18:5 (1994): 345–350.

Insulin Management: Blood Sugar Regulating Supplements

Broca, C., et al. "4-Hydroxyisoleucine: Experimental Evidence of Its Insulinotropic and Antidiabetic Properties." *Am J Physiol* 277:4 Part 1 (1999): E617–E623.

Docherty, J.P., et al. "A Double-blind, Placebo-controlled, Exploratory Trial of Chromium Picolinate in Atypical Depression: Effect on Carbohydrate Craving." *J Psychiatr Pract* 11:5 (2005): 302–314.

Fawcett, J.P., et al. "The Effect of Oral Vanadyl Sulfate on Body Composition and Performance in Weight-training Athletes." *Int J Sport Nutr* 6:4 (1996): 382–390.

Friedman, J.E., P.D. Neufer, and G.L. Dohm. "Regulation of Glycogen Resynthesis Following Exercise: Dietary Considerations." *Sports Med* 11:4 (1991): 232–243.

Grant, K.E., R.M. Chandler, A.L. Castle, and J.L. Ivy. "Chromium and Exercise Training: Effect on Obese Women." *Med Sci Sports Exercise* 29 (1997): 992–998.

Groff, J., S. Gropper, and S. Hunt. *Advanced Nutrition and Human Metabolism*, 2nd ed. St. Paul, MN: West Publishing, 1995.

Ikeda, Y. "The Clinical Study on the Water Extract of Leaves of *Lagerstroemia speciosa L* for Mild Cases of Diabetes Mellitus." (Pilot study.) Tokyo: Jikeikai University, 1998.

Jamieson, J., L. Dorman, and V. Marriot. *Growth Hormone: Reversing Human Aging Naturally*. East Canaan, CT: Safe Goods, 1997.

Klip, A., T. Ramal, D.A. Young, et al. "Insulin-induced Translocation of Glucose Transporters in Rat Hindlimb Muscles." *FEBS Lett* 224:1 (1987): 224–230.

Narayanan, C. "Pinitol-A New Anti-Diabetic Compound from the Leaves of Bougainvillea." *Curr Sci* 56:3 (1987): 139–141.

Newsholme, E.A., and A.R. Leech. *Biochemistry for the Medical Sciences*. New York: John Wiley & Sons, 1984, pp. 38–42, 312–330, 444–454.

Packer, L. "Antioxidant Properties of Lipoic Acid and Its Therapeutic Effects in Prevention of Diabetes Complications and Cataracts." *Annals NY Acad Sci* 738 (1994): 257–264.

Rodnick, K.J., E.J. Henriksen, D.E. James, et al. "Exercise Training, Glucose Transporters, and Glucose Transport in Rat Skeletal Muscles." *Am J Physiol* 262:1 (1992): C9–C14.

Wallberg-Henriksson, H., S.H. Constable, D.A. Young, et al. "Glucose Transport into Rat Skeletal Muscle: Interaction Between Exercise and Insulin." *J Appl Physiol* 65:2 (1998): 909–913.

Welihinda, J., et al. "Effect of *Momordica charantia* on the Glucose Tolerance in Maturity Onset Diabetes." *J Ethnopharmacol* 17:3 (1986): 277–282.

Wong, C.M., et al. "Insulin-like Molecules in *Momordica charantia* Seeds." *J Ethnopharmacol* 15:1 (1986): 107–117.

Cortisol Blocking

Brillon, D.J., B. Zheng, R.G. Campbell, and D.E. Matthews. "Effect of Cortisol on Energy Expenditure and Amino Acid Metabolism in Humans." *Am J Physiol* 268 (1995): E501–E513.

Burke, E., and T. Fahey. *Phosphatidylserine (PS): Promise for Athletic Performance*. New Canaan, CT: Keats Publishing, 1998.

Crook, T., et al. "Effects of Phosphatidylserine in Age-associated Memory Impairment." *Neurology* 41 (1991): 644–649.

Fahey, et al. "The Hormonal and Perceptive Effects of Phosphatidylserine Administration during Two Weeks of Resistive Exercise-induced Overtraining." *Biol Sport* 15 (1998): 135–144.

Griffin, J., and S. Ojeda. *Textbook of Endocrine Physiology,* 3rd ed. New York: Oxford University Press, 1996.

Monteleone, P., et al. "Blunting by Chronic Phosphatidylserine Administration of the Stress-induced Activation of the Hypothalamo-pituitary-adrenal Axis in Healthy Men." *Eur J Clin Pharamacol* 41 (1992): 385–388.

Monteleone, P., et al. "Effects of Phosphatidylserine on the Neuroendocrine Responses to Physical Stress in Humans." *Neuroendocrinology* 52 (1990): 243–248.

Palmieri, G., et al. "Double-blind Controlled Trial of Phosphatidylserine in Subjects with Senile Mental Deterioration." *Clin Trials J* 24 (1987): 73–83.

Simmons, P.S., J.M. Miles, J.E. Gerich, et al. "Increased Proteolysis: An Effect of Increases in Plasma Cortisol Within the Physiological Range." *J Clin Invest* 73 (1984): 412–420.

Hormone Modifiers

Argente, J., et al. "Growth Hormone–releasing Peptides: Clinical and Basic Aspects." *Horm Res* 46:4–5 (1996): 155–159.

Brilla, L.R., and V. Conte. "Effects of Zinc-Magnesium Formulation Increases Anabolic Hormones and Strength in Athletes." *Med Sci Sports Exer* 31:5 (1999): 483.

Di Luigi, L., et al. "Acute Amino Acids Supplementation Enhances Pituitary Responsiveness in Athletes." *Med Sci Sports Exerc* 31:12 (1999): 1748–1754.

Ghigo, E., et al. "Orally Active Growth Hormone Secretagogues: State of the Art and Clinical Perspectives." *Ann Med* 30:2 (1998): 159–168.

Gopal, K., et al. "Clinical Trial of Ethyl Acetate Extract of Gum Gugulu (Gugulipid) in Primary Hyperlipidemia." *J Assoc Physicians India* 34:4 (1986): 249–251.

Griffin, J., and S. Ojeda. *Textbook of Endocrine Physiology,* 3rd ed. New York: Oxford University Press, 1996.

Hofman, L.F. "Human Saliva as a Diagnostic Specimen." *J Nutr* 131:5 (2001): 1621S-1625S.

Jamieson, J., L. Dorman, and V. Marriot. *Growth Hormone: Reversing Human Aging Naturally.* East Canaan, CT: Safe Goods, 1997.

Kanaley, J., Weltman JY, Pieper KS, et al. "Cortisol and Growth Hormone Responses to Exercise at Different Times of the Day." *J Clin Endocrinol Metab* 86:6 (2001): 2881–2889.

Kelley, et al. "Energy Restriction and Immunocompetence in Overweight Women." *Nutr Res* 18:2 (1998): 159–169.

Lambert, M., et al. "Failure of Commercial Amino Acid Supplements to Increase Serum Growth Hormone Concentrations in Male Body-builders." *Int J Sport Nutr* 3:3 (1993): 298–305.

Le Bail, Jean-Christophe, et. al. "Chalcones are potent inhibitors of aromatase and 17 b-hydroxysteroid dehydrogenase activities." *Life Sciences* 68 (2001): 751–761.

Le Blanc J, et al. "Components of Postprandial Thermogenesis in Relation to Meal Frequency in Humans." *Can J Physiol Pharmacol* 71:12 (1993): 879–883.

Monteleone, P., et al. "Blunting by Chronic Phosphatidylserine Administration of the Stress-induced Activation of the Hypothalamo-pituitary-adrenal Axis in Healthy Men." *Eur J Clin Pharamacol* 41 (1992): 385–388.

Monteleone, P., et al. "Effects of Phosphatidylserine on the Neuroendocrine Responses to Physical Stress in Humans." *Neuroendocrinology* 52 (1990): 243–248.

Nazar, K., A.W. Zemba, B. Kruk, et al. "Phosphate Supplementation Prevents a Decrease of Triiodothyronine and Increases Resting Metabolic Rate during Low-energy Diet." *J Physiol Pharmacol* 47:2 (1996): 373–383.

Nityanand, S., et al. "Clinical Trials with Gugulipid: A New Hypolipidaemic Agent." *J Assoc Physicians India* 37:5 (1989): 323–328.

Volek, J., W. Kraemer, J. Bush, et al. "Testosterone and Cortisol in Relationship to Dietary Nutrients and Resistance Exercise." *J Appl Physiol* 82:1 (1997): 49–54.

Wankhede, S., et. al. "A double blind, randomized, placebo controlled human study on Testofen to evaluate its effect on muscle mass and free testosterone increase." Gencor Pacific (2006).

Weltman, A., et al. "Body Composition, Physical Exercise, Growth Hormone and Obesity." *Eat Weight Disord* 6:3 Suppl (2001): 28–37.

Joint Health and Repair

Cazzola, M., et al. "Oral Type II Collagen in the Treatment of Rheumatoid Arthritis: A Six-Month, Double-Blind Placebo-Controlled Study." *Clin Exp Rheumatol* 18:5 (2000): 571–577.

Drovanti, A., A.A. Bignamini, and A.L. Rovati. "Therapeutic Activity of Oral Glucosamine Sulfate in Osteoarthritis: A Placebo-Controlled, Double-Blind Investigation." *Clin Ther* 3:4 (1980): 260–272.

Hesslink, R., et al. "Cetylated Fatty Acids Improve Knee Function in Patients with Osteoarthritis." *J Rheumatol* 29:8 (2002): 1708–1712.

Mazieres, B., et al. "Le Chondroitin Sulfate Dayns le Traitment de la Gonarthose et de la Coxarthrose." *Rev Rheum Mal Osteoartic* 59:7–8 (1992): 466–472.

Moskowitz, R.W. "Role of Collagen Hydrolysate in Bone and Joint Disease." *Semin Arthritis Rheum* 30:2 (2000): 87–99.

Parcell, S. "Sulfur in Human Nutrition and Applications in Medicine." *Altern Med Rev* 7:1 (2002): 22–44.

Pipitone, V.R. "Chondroprotection with Chondroitin Sulfate." *Drugs Exp Clin Res* 17:1 (1991): 3–7.

Reginster, J.Y., et al. "Long-Term Effects of Glucosamine Sulphate on Osteoarthritis Progression: A Randomised, Placebo-Controlled Clinical Trial." *The Lancet* 357:9252 (2001): 251–256.

Simanek, V., et al. "The Efficacy of Glucosamine and Chondroitin Sulfate in the Treatment of Osteoarthritis: Are These Saccharides Drugs or Nutraceuticals?" *Biomed Pap Med Fac Univ Palacky Olomouc Czech Repub* 149:1 (2005): 51–56.

Tapadinhas, M.J., et al. "Oral Glucosamine Sulfate in the Management of Arthrosis: Report on a Multi-Centre Open Investigation in Portugal." *Pharmatherapeutica* 3 (1982): 157–168.

Theodosakis, J., et al. *The Arthritis Cure.* New York: St. Martin's Press, 1997.

Trentham, D.E., et al. "Effects of Oral Administration of Type II Collagen on Rheumatoid Arthritis." *Science* 261:5129 (1993): 1727–1730.

Supplement Timing

Alessio, H.M., et al. "Exercise-induced Oxidative Stress Before and After Vitamin C Supplementation." *Int J Sport Nutr* 7:1 (1997): 1–9.

Balakrishnan, S.D., and C.V. Anuradha. "Exercise, Depletion of Antioxidants and Antioxidant Manipulation." *Cell Biochem Funct* 16:4 (1998): 269–275.

Bell, D.G., et al. "Effect of Caffeine and Ephedrine Ingestion on Anaerobic Exercise Performance." *Med Sci Sports Exerc* 33:8 (2001): 1399–1403.

Bloomer, R.J., et al. "Effects of Meal Form and Composition on Plasma Testosterone, Cortisol, and Insulin Following Resistance Exercise." *Int J Sport Nutr Exerc Metab* 10:4 (2000): 415–424.

Brilla, L.R., and V. Conte. "Effects of Zinc-Magnesium Formulation Increases Anabolic Hormones and Strength in Athletes." *Med Sci Sports Exer* 31:5 (1999): 483.

Brilla, L.R., and T.F. Haley. "Effect of Magnesium Supplementation on Strength Training in Humans." *J Amer Coll Nutr* 11:3 (1992): 326–329.

Broca, C., et al. "4-Hydroxyisoleucine: Experimental Evidence of its Insulinotropic and Antidiabetic Properties." *Am J Physiol* 277:4 Part 1 (1999): E617–E623.

Costill, D.L., and M. Hargreaves. "Carbohydrate Nutrition and Fatigue." *Sports Med* 13:2 (1992): 86–92.

Crawford, V., et al. "Effects of Niacin-bound Chromium Supplementation on Body Composition in Overweight African-American Women." *Diabetes Obes Metab* 1:6 (1999): 331–337.

Doi, T., et al. "New Approach for Weight Reduction by a Combination of Diet, Light Resistance Exercise and the Timing of Ingesting a Protein Supplement." *Asia Pac J Clin Nutr* 10:3 (2001): 226–232.

Esmarck, B., et al. "Timing of Postexercise Protein Intake is Important for Muscle Hypertrophy with Resistance Training in Elderly Humans." *J Physiol* 15 (2001): 301–311.

Fahey, et al. "The Hormonal and Perceptive Effects of Phosphatidylserine Administration during Two Weeks of Resistive Exercise-induced Overtraining." *Biol Sport* 15 (1998): 135–144.

Goss, F., et al. "Effect of Potassium Phosphate Supplementation on Perceptual and Physiological Responses to Maximal Graded Exercise." *Int J Sport Nutr Exerc Metab* 11:1 (2001): 53–62.

Graham, T. "Caffeine and Exercise: Metabolism, Endurance, and Performance." *Sports Med* 31:11 (2001): 785–807.

Griffiths, R.D. "Glutamine: Establishing Clinical Indications." *Curr Opin Clin Nutr Metab Care* 2:2 (1999): 177–182.

Hargreaves, M. "Pre-exercise Nutritional Strategies: Effects on Metabolism and Performance." *Can J Appl Physiol* 26 (2001): S64–S70.

Ivy, J.L. "Dietary Strategies to Promote Glycogen Synthesis after Exercise." *Can J Appl Physiol* 26 (2001): S236–S245.

Kraemer, W.J., et al. "Hormonal Responses to Consecutive Days of Heavy-resistance Exercise With or Without Nutritional Supplementation." *J Appl Physiol* 85:4 (1998): 1544–1555.

Liu, Z., L.A. Jahn, W. Long, et al. "Branched Chain Amino Acids Activate Messenger Ribonucleic Acid Translation Regulatory Proteins in Human Skeletal Muscle, and Glucocorticoids Blunt This Action." *J Clin Endocrinol Metab* 86:5 (2001): 2136–2143.

Mittleman, K.D., et al. "Branched-chain Amino Acids Prolong Exercise during Heat Stress in Men and Women." *Med Sci Sports Exerc* 30:1 (1998): 83–91.

Nieman, D.C. "Exercise Immunology: Nutritional Countermeasures." *Can J Appl Physiol* 26 (2001): S45–S55.

Panton, L.B., et al. "Nutritional Supplementation of the Leucine Metabolite HMB during Resistance Training." *Nutrition* 16 (2000): 734–739.

Peters, E.M., R. Anderson, D.C. Nieman, et al. "Vitamin C Supplementation Attenuates the Increases in Circulating Cortisol, Adrenaline and Anti-inflammatory Polypeptides Following Ultramarathon Running." *Int J Sports Med* 22:7 (2001): 537–543.

Peters, E.M., et al. "Attenuation of Increase in Circulating Cortisol and Enhancement of the Acute Phase Protein Response in Vitamin C–Supplemented Ultramarathoners." *Int J Sports Med* 22:2 (2001): 120–126.

Roy, B.D., et al. "Effect of Glucose Supplement Timing on Protein Metabolism after Resistance Training." *J Appl Physiol* 82:6 (1997): 1882–1888.

Schroder, H., et al. "Effects of Alpha-tocopherol, Beta-carotene and Ascorbic Acid on Oxidative, Hormonal and Enzymatic Exercise Stress Markers in Habitual Training Activity of Professional Basketball Players." *Eur J Nutr* 40:4 (2001): 178–184.

Schroder, H., et al. "Nutrition Antioxidant Status and Oxidative Stress in Professional Basketball Players: Effects of a Three-compound Antioxidative Supplement." *Int J Sports Med* 21:2 (2000): 146–150.

Sen, C.K. "Antioxidants in Exercise Nutrition." *Sports Med* 31:13 (2001): 891–908.

Sen, C.K. "Update on Thiol Status and Supplements in Physical Exercise." *Can J Appl Physiol* 26 (2001): S4–S12.

Terjung, R.L., et al. "The Physiological and Health Effects of Oral Creatine Supplementation." *Med Sci Sports Exerc* 32.3 (2000): 706–717.

Van Hall, G., W.H. Saris, P.A. van de Schoor, and A.J. Wagenmakers. "The Effect of Free Glutamine and Peptide Ingestion on the Rate of Muscle Glycogen Resynthesis in Man." *Int J Sports Med* 21:1 (2000): 25–30.

Volek, J.S., et al. "L-carnitine L-tartrate Supplementation Favorably Effects Markers of Recovery from Exercise Stress." *Am J Physiol Endocrinol Metab* 282:2 (2002): E474–E482.

Vukovich, M.D., et al. "Effect of Beta-hydroxy-beta-methylbutyrate on the Outset of Blood Lactate Accumulation and VO_2 Peak in Endurance Trained Cyclists." *J Strength Cond Res* 15:4 (2001): 491–497.

Wenos, D.L., and H.K. Amato. "Weight Cycling Alters Muscular Strength and Endurance, Ratings of Perceived Exertion, and Total Body Water in College Wrestlers." *Percept Motor Skills* 87:3 Part 1 (1998): 975–978.

Wolfe, R.R. "Effects of Amino Acid Intake on Anabolic Processes." *Can J Appl Physiol* 26:Suppl (2001): S220–S227.

Yaspelkis, B.B. 3rd, and Ivy, J.L. "The Effect of a Carbohydrate-Arginine Supplement on Postexercise Carbohydrate Metabolism." *Int J Sport Nutr* 9:3 (1999): 241–250.

Index

About the Authors

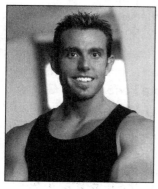

Stephen Adelé has been helping individuals from all walks of life create measurable results in their physiques and performance over the last fifteen years, and has become a respected authority at the age of 35. He has published numerous articles for magazines around the world, been quoted in several trade publications, appeared on radio and television shows, conducted seminars around the globe, and is the CEO of the prestigious supplement manufacturer, iSatori Technologies (isatoritech.com).

Stephen now also shares his insights, expertise, and inside connections in two of the fastest growing publications in the industry, *Real SOLUTIONS* email newsletter and *Real SOLUTIONS* magazine (realsolutionsmag.com), and has authored several best-selling consumers' guides, including: *The 21-Day Ultimate Energy Plan, The Lean System Success Plan, The Carnosine Breakthrough,* and *MAXIMUM GROWTH, Volumes I & II.*

Over the years, Stephen's philosophy has remained unchanged: "The greatest gift you can give yourself is the gift of a strong mind, which can yield extraordinary dividends in the form of a stronger, healthier, and more energetic body."

Stephen resides in Golden, Colorado where he lives with his wife and three girls. You can learn more about Stephen, subscribe to his monthly newsletter, and receive a bonus report entitled *7 Never-Before-Told Secrets Everyone Should Know Before Buying Supplements* by visiting RealSolutionsMag.com.

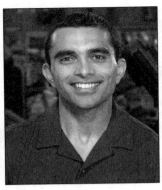

Rehan Jalali is President of the Beverly Hills, California-based Supplement Research Foundation (www.tsrf.com). He is a nationally recognized Certified Sports Nutritionist (C.S.N.) who has developed over one hundred cutting-edge products for the dietary supplement industry. His clients include Oscar® winning actors, Emmy® award winning TV stars, and Grammy® winning musicians. He has developed advanced customized nutrition and supplementation programs for actors getting ready for movie roles, musicians preparing for videos, and celebrities peaking for appearances including award shows. He has over 250 nationally and internationally published articles on nutrition and supplementation.

Rehan has worked with many Olympic and professional athletes including Gold medalists. Long considered an authority on sports nutrition, Rehan is the author of *The Six Pack Diet Plan*, *The Ultimate Performance Guide to Fitness Success*, and co-author of *The Bodybuilding Supplement Guide*. He is host of the supplement segment on the weekly Canadian TV show *The Art of Building Bodies*.

He is a nationally published scientific writer, monthly columnist, and model who has appeared in *Newsweek*, *US Weekly*, *Life&Style*, *InTouch*, *Men's Health*, *Muscle and Fitness*, *Men's Fitness*, *Ironman Magazine*, *Physical*, *Let's Live*, *SLY*, *Maximum Fitness*, *MuscleMag International*, *Nirvana*, *Inside Fitness*, *Health Supplement Retailer*, *Vitamin Retailer*, *Oxygen*, *Muscle Media*, *Hydrate*, *Adrenaline*, *Whole Foods Magazine*, *Grappling*, *Mind and Muscle Power*, *Real Solutions*, *Personal Fitness Professional*, *Health Products Business*, *Olympian's News*, *The Washington Post*, *The Orange County Register*, the *Houston Chronicle*, *Angeleno*, *Human Performance*, *Muscle News*, *Muscle&Body*, *Pumped*, Drkoop.com, thinkmuscle.com, and Mesomorphosis.com among others.

Rehan is also a natural bodybuilder who has appeared on ESPN and CBS. He has held numerous bodybuilding titles, including Mr. Texas and the Ironman Naturally Bodybuilding Champion. He is a member of the American Medical Writer's Association.